P9-CIU-604

Walker S. Carlos Poston II, PhD
C. Keith Haddock, PhD
Editors

Food as a Drug

Food as a Drug has been co-published simultaneously as *Drugs & Society,* Volume 15, Numbers 1/2 1999.

Pre-Publication
REVIEWS,
COMMENTARIES,
EVALUATIONS . . .

"**T**his volume by Poston and Haddock provides a synthesis of a controversial and understudied topic in a manner that is both scholarly and accessible. Its strength is the variety of approaches taken to examining food as a drug including pharmacologic, psychological, legal, nutritional and cultural. In addition to reviewing the evidence from each of these areas, several articles review the validity of an addictions model in the treatment of eating disorders and obesity. *Food as a Drug* will serve as a useful resource for clinicians and researchers alike. I highly recommend it."

Gary D. Foster, PhD
Clinical Director
Weight and Eating Disorders Program
University of Pennsylvania
School of Medicine
Philadelphia

Food as a Drug

Food as a Drug has been co-published simultaneously as *Drugs & Society*, Volume 15, Numbers 1/2 1999.

The Drugs & Society Monographic *"Separates"*

Below is a list of "separates," which in serials librarianship means a special issue simultaneously published as a special journal issue or double-issue *and* as a "separate" hardbound monograph. (This is a format which we also call a "DocuSerial.")

"Separates" are published because specialized libraries or professionals may wish to purchase a specific thematic issue by itself in a format which can be separately cataloged and shelved, as opposed to purchasing the journal on an on-going basis. Faculty members may also more easily consider a "separate" for classroom adoption.

"Separates" are carefully classified separately with the major book jobbers so that the journal tie-in can be noted on new book order slips to avoid duplicate purchasing.

You may wish to visit Haworth's website at . . .

http://www.haworthpressinc.com

. . . to search our online catalog for complete tables of contents of these separates and related publications.

You may also call 1-800-HAWORTH (outside US/Canada: 607-722-5857), or Fax 1-800-895-0582 (outside US/Canada: 607-771-0012), or e-mail at:

getinfo@haworthpressinc.com

Food as a Drug, edited by Walker S. Carlos Poston II, PhD, and C. Keith Haddock, PhD (Vol. 15, No. 1/2, 1999). *This book provides a synthesis of a controversial and understudied topic. . . . Its strength is in the variety of approaches taken to examining food as a drug . . . serves as a useful resource for clinicians and researchers alike. (Gary D. Foster, PhD, Clinical Director, Weight and Eating Disorders Program, University of Pennsylvania, School of Medicine, Philadelphia)*

Conducting Drug Abuse Research with Minority Populations: Advances and Issues, edited by Mario R. De La Rosa, PhD, Bernard Segal, PhD, and Richard Lopez, PhD (Vol. 14, No. 1/2, 1998). *Provides you with an excellent overview of the most important issues that need to be taken into account when conducting drug abuse research within minority populations.*

Women and Substance Abuse: Gender Transparency, edited by Sally J. Stevens, PhD, and Harry K. Wexler, PhD (Vol. 13, No. 1/2, 1998). *"The findings presented in this book are timely and comprehensive and indicate the devastating societal, medical and economic consequences of substance abuse. . . .* Women and Substance Abuse *is a wake-up call for all." (Linda B. Cottler, PhD, Associate Professor of Epidemiology in Psychiatry, Washington University School of Medicine, St. Louis, Missouri)*

Substance Abuse Prevention in Multicultural Communities, edited by Jeanette Valentine, PhD, Judith A. De Jong, PhD, and Nancy J. Kennedy, DrPH (Vol. 12, No. 1/2, 1998). *"Makes significant contributions to evaluation methodology as well as to prevention theory and research." (Lonnie R. Sherrod, PhD, Executive Vice President, William T. Grant Foundation, New York, New York)*

Sociocultural Perspectives on Volatile Solvent Use, edited by Fred Beauvais, PhD, and Joseph E. Trimble, PhD (Vol. 10, No. 1/2, 1997). *Presents groundbreaking, vital information about the problem of solvent abuse among American Indian and Alaskan Native youth.*

Multicultural AIDS Prevention Programs, edited by Robert T. Trotter II (Vol. 9, No. 1/2, 1996). *"Provides extremely important background for any ongoing research that involves HIV and drug prevention efforts. . . . A recommended book for all academic, medical, and large public libraries." (AIDS Book Review Journal)*

Prevention Practice in Substance Abuse, edited by Carl G. Leukefeld, DSW, and Richard R. Clayton, PhD (Vol. 8, No. 3/4, 1995). *"An authoritative state-of-the-art compendium, covering a remarkably wide range of modern efforts on the theory and practice of substance abuse prevention. . . . Highly recommended." (Addiction)*

Innovations in Alcoholism Treatment: State of the Art Reviews and Their Implications for Clinical Practice, edited by Gerard J. Connors, PhD (Vol. 8, No. 1, 1994). *"Distills a remarkable amount of information into a very small space and is, furthermore, an easy read as well as a useful reference."* (*Science Books & Films*)

AIDS and Community-Based Drug Intervention Programs: Evaluation and Outreach, edited by Dennis G. Fisher, PhD, and Richard Needle, PhD (Vol. 7, No. 3/4, 1993). *"An excellent resource for AIDS prevention researchers and provides fine examples of community-based intervention."* (*David P. Mackinnon, PhD, Assistant Professor, Department of Psychology, Arizona State University*)

Drug Use in Rural American Communities, edited by Ruth W. Edwards, PhD (Vol. 7, No. 1/2, 1993). *"This single source provides access to the last 15 years of research, treatment, and policymaking in ths increasingly important area."* (*William Alex McIntosh, PhD, Department of Sociology, Texas A & M University*)

Ethnic and Multicultural Drug Abuse: Perspectives on Current Research, edited by Joseph E. Trimble, PhD, Catherine S. Bolek, MS, and Steve J. Niemcryk, PhD (Vol. 6, No. 1/2/ 3/4, 1993). *"Communicate detailed information, report multivariate statistical analyses, and provide extensive reference lists."* (*Contemporary Psychology*)

Homelessness and Drinking: A Study of a Street Population, edited by Bernard Segal, PhD (Vol. 5, No. 3/4, 1992). *"Will appeal to serious students of homelessness, particularly those interested in alcohol and drug abuse."* (*Journal of Studies on Alcohol*)

AIDS and Alcohol/Drug Abuse: Psychosocial Research, edited by Dennis G. Fisher, PhD (Vol. 5, No. 1/2, 1991). *"AIDS and its curious relationship with substance abuse is explored by drug abuse researchers in this pertinent book. In a poignantly written selection on one of the book's major focuses, experts discuss some of the pitfalls that have befallen researchers doing AIDS research on minorities."* (*Lambda Book Report*)

Addictive Disorders in Arctic Climates: Theory, Research, and Practice at the Novosibirsk Institute, edited by Bernard Segal, PhD, and Caesar P. Korolenko, MD (Vol. 4, No. 3/4, 1991). *"The interplay of biological and psychological factors in addiction against a background of issues . . . are of crucial concern in understanding the development of addictions."* (*British Journal of Addiction*)

Drug-Taking Behavior Among School-Aged Youth: The Alaska Experience and Comparisons with Lower-48 States, edited by Bernard Segal, PhD (Vol. 4, No. 1/2, 1990). *"An interesting, easily read and easily understood text that would be relevant for any and all treatment professionals, in particular those who deal in the area of adolescent drug abuse."* (*Criminal Justice Review*)

Current Issues in Alcohol/Drug Studies, edited by Edith S. Lisansky Gomberg, PhD (Vol. 3, No. 3/4, 1990). *"A fine collection of reasonable, provocative, and thoughtful papers. In all, the book provides much needed clear thinking about very complex problems that are clouded in controversy and confusion."* (*Robert Straus, PhD, Professor, Department of Behavioral Science, College of Medicine, University of Kentucky; Author of* Drinking in College *(Yale University Press, 1953),* Escape From Custody *(Harper & Row, 1974), and* Alcohol and Society *(1973))*

Perspectives on Adolescent Drug Use, edited by Bernard Segal, PhD (Vol. 3, No. 1/2, 1989). *"This is an important and very current summary collection of what is known about adolescent drug involvement."* (*Robert A. Zucker, PhD, Professor of Psychology, Michigan State University*)

Alcoholism Etiology and Treatment: Issues for Theory and Practice, edited by Bernard Segal, PhD (Vol. 2, No. 3/4, 1989). *"Anyone involved in alcohol treatment research should be aware of alternatives to the disease concept of alcoholism, and there is no better way to learn than by reading this book."* (*American Journal of Psychotherapy, April 1991*)

Research Strategies in Alcoholism Treatment, edited by Dan J. Lettieri, PhD (Vol. 2, No. 2, 1989). *This book highlights the practical issues inherent in planning and conducting alcohol treatment assessment research.*

Perspectives on Person-Environment Interaction and Drug-Taking Behavior, edited by Bernard Segal, PhD (Vol. 2, No. 1, 1988). *A comprehensive review of the interactionist approach to drug use from both a theoretical and applied perspective.*

Drug Use and Psychological Theory, edited by S. W. Sadava, PhD (Vol. 1, No. 4, 1987). *An exciting exploration of the linkages between drug use and other patterns of behavior.*

Moderation as a Goal or Outcome of Treatment for Alcohol Problems: A Dialogue, edited by Mark B. Sobell, PhD, and Linda C. Sobell, PhD (Vol. 1, No. 2/3, 1987). *"Of value to treatment professionals and clinical scientists, students, and others interested in learning about the evolving conceptualizations of alcohol problems." (Contemporary Psychology)*

Perspectives on Drug Use in the United States, edited by Bernard Segal, PhD (Vol. 1, No. 1, 1986). *Perceptive critical analyses of areas of concern within the field that have important implications for both research endeavors and clinical intervention.*

OKANAGAN UNIVERSITY COLLEGE
LIBRARY
BRITISH COLUMBIA

Food as a Drug

Walker S. Carlos Poston II, PhD
C. Keith Haddock, PhD
Editors

Food as a Drug has been co-published simultaneously as *Drugs & Society*, Volume 15, Numbers 1/2 1999.

The Haworth Press, Inc.
New York • London • Oxford

Food as a Drug has been co-published simultaneously as *Drugs & Society* ™ , Volume 15, Numbers 1/2 1999.

© 2000 by The Haworth Press, Inc. All rights reserved. No part of this work may be reproduced or utilized in any form or by any means, electronic or mechanical, including photocopying, microfilm and recording, or by any information storage and retrieval system, without permission in writing from the publisher. Printed in the United States of America.

The development, preparation, and publication of this work has been undertaken with great care. However, the publisher, employees, editors, and agents of The Haworth Press and all imprints of The Haworth Press, Inc., including The Haworth Medical Press® and Pharmaceutical Products Press®, are not responsible for any errors contained herein or for consequences that may ensue from use of materials or information contained in this work. Opinions expressed by the author(s) are not necessarily those of The Haworth Press, Inc.

The Haworth Press, Inc., 10 Alice Street, Binghamton, NY 13904-1580 USA

Library of Congress Cataloging-in-Publication Data

Food as a Drug / Walker S. Carlos Poston II, C. Keith Haddock, editors.
    p.cm.
   "Co-published simultaneously as Drugs & society, volume 15, numbers 1/2 1999."
   Includes bibliographical references and index.
   ISBN 0-7890-0959-5 (alk. paper) -- ISBN 0-7890-0977-3 (pbk. : alk. paper)
   1. Compulsive eating. 2. Eating disorders. 3. Functional foods. 4. Dietary supplements.
I. Poston, Walker S. Carlos, II. II. Haddock, C. Keith.
RC552.C65 .F66 2000
616.85'26--dc21
                                              99-088150

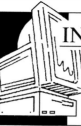

INDEXING & ABSTRACTING

Contributions to this publication are selectively indexed or abstracted in print, electronic, online, or CD-ROM version(s) of the reference tools and information services listed below. This list is current as of the copyright date of this publication. See the end of this section for additional notes.

- *Abstracts in Anthropology*

- *Academic Abstracts/CD-ROM*

- *ADDICTION ABSTRACTS*

- *ALCONLINE Database*

- *Applied Social Sciences Index & Abstracts (ASSIA) (Online: ASSI via Data-Star) (CDRom: ASSIA Plus)*

- *Brown University Digest of Addiction Theory and Application, The (DATA Newsletter)*

- *BUBL Information Service: An Internet-based Information Service for the UK higher education community <URL: http://bubl.ac.uk/>*

- *Cambridge Scientific Abstracts*

- *Child Development Abstracts & Bibliography*

- *CNPIEC Reference Guide: Chinese National Directory of Foreign Periodicals*

- *Criminal Justice Abstracts*

- *Criminal Justice Periodical Index*

- *EMBASE/Excerpta Medica Secondary Publishing Division*

- *Family Studies Database (online and CD/ROM)*

- *HealthPromis*

- *Health Source: Indexing & Abstracting of 160 selected health related journals, updated monthly: EBSCO Publishing*

- *Health Source Plus: expanded version of "Health Source": EBSCO Publishing*

- *Human Resources Abstracts (HRA)*

(continued)

- *IBZ International Bibliography of Periodical Literature*
- *Index to Periodical Articles Related to Law*
- *International Pharmaceutical Abstracts*
- *International Political Science Abstracts/Documentation Politique Internationale*
- *Mental Health Abstracts (online through DIALOG)*
- *National Center for Chronic Disease Prevention & Health Promotion (NCCDPHP)*
- *National Criminal Justice Reference Service*
- *NIAAA Alcohol & Alcohol Problems Science Database (ETOH)*
- *PAIS (Public Affairs Information Service) NYC www.pais.org*
- *Personnel Management Abstracts*
- *Psychological Abstracts (PsycINFO)*
- *Referativnyi Zhurnal (Abstracts Journal of the All-Russian Institute of Scientific and Technical Information)*
- *Sage Family Studies Abstracts (SFSA)*
- *Social Services Abstracts*
- *Social Sciences Index (from Volume 1 & continuing)*
- *Social Work Abstracts*
- *Sociological Abstracts (SA)*
- *SOMED (social medicine) Database*
- *Spanish Technical Information System on Drug Abuse Prevention "Sistema de Informacion Tecnica Sobre Prevencion del Abuso de Drogas, IDEA-Prevencion"*
- *SPORT Discus*
- *Violence and Abuse Abstracts: A Review of Current Literature on Interpersonal Violence (VAA)*

(continued)

Special Bibliographic Notes related to special journal issues (separates) and indexing/abstracting:

- indexing/abstracting services in this list will also cover material in any "separate" that is co-published simultaneously with Haworth's special thematic journal issue or DocuSerial. Indexing/abstracting usually covers material at the article/chapter level.
- monographic co-editions are intended for either non-subscribers or libraries which intend to purchase a second copy for their circulating collections.
- monographic co-editions are reported to all jobbers/wholesalers/approval plans. The source journal is listed as the "series" to assist the prevention of duplicate purchasing in the same manner utilized for books-in-series.
- to facilitate user/access services all indexing/abstracting services are encouraged to utilize the co-indexing entry note indicated at the bottom of the first page of each article/chapter/contribution.
- this is intended to assist a library user of any reference tool (whether print, electronic, online, or CD-ROM) to locate the monographic version if the library has purchased this version but not a subscription to the source journal.
- individual articles/chapters in any Haworth publication are also available through the Haworth Document Delivery Service (HDDS).

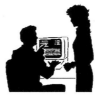

ALL HAWORTH BOOKS AND JOURNALS
ARE PRINTED ON CERTIFIED
ACID-FREE PAPER

Food as a Drug

CONTENTS

Preface   xv

Pharmacological Properties of Foods and Nutrients   1
Jane V. White, PhD, RD
Rebecca S. Reeves, DrPH, RD

The Effects of Food on Mood and Behavior: Implications
for the Addictions Model of Obesity and Eating Disorders   17
C. Keith Haddock, PhD
Patricia L. Dill, MS

Medicinal Foods: Cross-Cultural Perspectives   49
Chu-Huang Chen, MD, PhD
Devin C. Volding, MSW

Legal and Regulatory Perspectives on Dietary Supplements
and Foods   65
Walker S. Carlos Poston II, PhD
Laurie Fan, MBA
Rich Rakowski, PharmD
Martin Ericsson, MD, PhD
Christopher C. Bunn, MS
John P. Foreyt, PhD

Eating Disorders and Addiction   87
G. Terence Wilson, PhD

Etiology and Treatment of Obesity in Adults and Children:
Implications for the Addiction Model   103
Risa J. Stein, PhD
Kristin Koetting O'Byrne, BA
Richard R. Suminski, PhD, MPH
C. Keith Haddock, PhD

Inability to Control Eating: Addiction to Food or Normal
Response to Abnormal Environment?   123
G. Ken Goodrick, PhD

Food as a Drug: Conclusions   141
   C. Keith Haddock, PhD
   Walker S. Carlos Poston II, PhD

Index   147

ABOUT THE EDITORS

Walker S. Carlos Poston II, PhD, is Assistant Professor in the Department of Medicine and the Behavioral Medicine Research Center at Baylor College of Medicine. He is a study section member in Behavioral Science and Epidemiology research in the U.S. Army Medical Research & Material Command Breast Cancer Research Program and the American Heart Association, Texas Affiliated. Dr. Poston has been a consultant to the American Institute of Biological Sciences in the area of behavioral interventions for chronic medical conditions and a consultant on disability and rehabilition to the United States Coast Guard Disability Adjudication Office. He has been a visiting scholar at the Karolinska Institute in Sweden. Dr. Poston is an active member in several professional societies including the American Psychological Association and the Society of Behavioral Medicine.

C. Keith Haddock, PhD, is Assistant Professor of Psychology and Medicine at the University of Missouri–Kansas City, and Co-Director of Behavioral Cardiology at the Mid America Heart Institute. Dr. Haddock is an active member of the American Psychological Association (APA), the Division of Health Psychology of the APA, the Society of Air Force Clinical Psychologists, the Society of Behavioral Medicine, and the Society for Research on Nicotine and Tobacco. He is a Captain in the U.S. Air Force reserves and is the Chief of Mental Health Services for the 442nd Fighter Wing, Whiteman AFB, Missouri. Dr. Haddock's research has been funded by both state and national granting agencies, and he has received numerous awards including a president's citation from the Society of Behavioral Medicine.

Preface

Why should anyone consider food to be a drug? Food is necessary to human survival and yet some individuals seem to have significant difficulties controlling their intake. For example, overweight and obesity are the most significant public health problems in the U.S. and many other industrialized nations (NIH/NHLBI, 1998; WHO, 1998). The age-adjusted prevalence of overweight and obesity, defined as a body mass index (BMI) $\geq$ 25 and < 30 BMI $\geq$ 30 is 32.6% and 22.3% in the U.S., respectively (NIH/NHLBI, 1998). While the prevalence of obesity has been increasing at alarming rates, cures have remained elusive. Similarly, the rates for eating disorders (i.e., anorexia, bulimia, and binge eating disorder) seem to have increased in the past 10 to 20 years, particularly among women ages 15 to 25 (Ash & Piazza, 1995; Edwards & Kerry, 1993; Vandereycken & Hoek, 1992). Eating disorders occur primarily in females (APA, 1994). The increases have coincided with a doubling over 20 years in the percentage of women who report negative body image attitudes (Berscheid, Walster, & Bohrnstedt, 1973; Cash & Henry, 1995).

Obesity and eating disorders extract tremendous societal and personal costs in the forms of increased risk for disease and death, health care costs associated with long-term treatment and, given their multifactorial nature, many experts recognize them as chronic diseases that require long-term, multidisciplinary management (Crisp, Callender, Halek, & Hsu, 1992; Howlett, McClelland, & Crisp, 1995; Hsu, 1995; Keller, Herzog, Lavori, Bradburn, & Mahoney, 1992; Kirschenbaum

The authors' work on this collection was partially supported by a Minority Scientist Development Award from the American Heart Association and with funds contributed by the AHA, Puerto Rico Affiliate and a faculty research grant from the University of Missouri-Kansas City.

[Haworth indexing entry note]: "Preface." Poston II, Walker S. Carlos, and C. Keith Haddock. Published in *Food as a Drug* (ed: Walker S. Carlos Poston II, and C. Keith Haddock) The Haworth Press, Inc., 2000, pp. xv-xix. Single or multiple copies of this article are available for a fee from The Haworth Document Delivery Service [1-800-342-9678, 9:00 a.m. - 5:00 p.m. (EST). E-mail address: getinfo@haworthpressinc.com].

© 2000 by The Haworth Press, Inc. All rights reserved.

& Fitzgibbon, 1995; NIH/NHLBI, 1998). Given their chronicity and intractability, it is not surprising that some writers in both the professional and popular literature have concluded that they are addictive disorders and that some foods might have addictive properties that trigger compulsive eating behaviors in affected individuals (Davis & Claridge, 1998; Heller & Heller, 1994; Parham, 1995; Sheppard, 1993; Wurtman, 1996).

While the explanations vary about how foods might be addictive, have drug-like effects, or might trigger addictive behaviors, and several neurobiological hypotheses for obesity and eating disorders have been explored, no definitive answers have been found (Ericsson, Poston, & Foreyt, 1996). This has not stemmed the popularity of food addiction models for these disorders, particularly in the popular press. Thus, this volume provides reviews of relevant topics including whether foods have pharmacological properties, diet and behavior relationships, cross-cultural perspectives on the use of foods for medicinal purposes, and regulatory perspectives on drugs, foods, and nutritional supplements. The first contribution by White and Reeves (2000) provides an excellent review of the evidence on whether foods, or more specifically, macronutrients, have pharmacological properties. Haddock and Dill (2000) review the evidence for diet-behavior relationships, with a specific focus on sugar, the effects of food additives on childrens' behavioral disorders (e.g., attention deficit and hyperactivity) and the role of diet on serotonin, carbohydrate craving, and depression. Chen and Volding (2000) review the historical and modern uses of foods as medicines in different cultures. Next, Poston and colleagues (2000) provide an overview of the legal and regulatory definitions and status of dietary/nutritional supplements, a specific legal category that includes vitamins, minerals, tissue extracts, amino acids and protein products, and herbal preparations.

In the latter part of this volume, several authors provide different perspectives on the question of whether obesity, anorexia, bulimia, and binge eating are addictive disorders and how well the addictions model fits these disorders. For example, Stein and her colleagues (2000) review the obesity treatment outcome literature and discuss their implications for addictions approaches to obesity. Wilson (2000) discusses conceptual problems with the addictions model when it is applied to eating disorders and the dearth of supportive empirical evidence for the carbohydrate craving hypothesis, as well as other addictions oriented models. Finally, Goodrick (2000) examines the phenomenological, psychological, and physiological correlates of overeating and discusses how foods may be used to alleviate negative mood states and potentiate compulsive eating after restrictive dieting. In addition, he notes that although compulsive eating may not fit an addictions model, the lack of self-control over food experienced by many eating-disordered and obese individuals has implications for treatment programs and health policy.

We would like to thank Dr. Segal for soliciting this collection on *Food as a Drug* and allowing us to present this important topic. We feel that this is an important subject because of the increasing recognition that obesity and eating disorders are chronic and difficult to treat. Current research provides few answers to questions about their etiology or optimal management. All of the contributions were solicited from colleagues with expertise in the obesity and eating disorders fields. In addition, all of the contributions were peer-reviewed by two reviewers to improve their content, organization, and readability. We feel that these articles make an important contribution to the ongoing debate about the value of the addictions model for obesity and eating disorders, as well as addressing important issues about the nature of food as a potentially addictive substance.

Walker S. Carlos Poston II, PhD
C. Keith Haddock, PhD

REFERENCES

American Psychiatric Association (APA). (1994). *Diagnostic and statistical manual of mental disorders* (4th ed.). Washington, DC: Author.

Ash, J. B., & Piazza, E. (1995). Changing symptomatology in eating disorders. *International Journal of Eating Disorders, 18,* 27-38.

Berscheid, E., Walster, E., & Bohrnstedt, G. (1973). Body image. The happy American body: A survey report. *Psychology Today, 7,* 119-131.

Cash, T. F., & Henry, P. E. (1995). Women's body images: The results of a national survey in the U.S.A. *Sex Roles, 33,* 19-28.

Chen, C. H., & Volding, D. C. (2000). Medicinal foods: Cross-cultural perspectives. In Poston, W. S. C. & Haddock C. K. (Eds.), *Food as a drug* (pp. 49-64). New York, NY: The Haworth Press, Inc.

Crisp, A. H. (1988). Some possible approaches to prevention of eating and body weight/shape disorders, with particular reference to anorexia nervosa. *International Journal of Eating Disorders, 7,* 1-17.

Davis, C., & Claridge, G. (1998). The eating disorder as addiction: A psychobiological perspective. *Addictive Behaviors*, *23*, 463-475.

Edwards, M. D., & Kerry I. (1993). Obesity, anorexia, and bulimia. *Clinical Nutrition*, *77*, 899-909.

Ericsson, M., Poston, W. S. C., & Foreyt, J. P. (1996). Common biological pathways in eating disorders and obesity. *Addictive Behaviors*, *21*, 733-743.

Goodrick, G. K. (2000). Inability to control eating: Addiction to food or normal response to abnormal environment? In Poston, W. S. C. & Haddock C. K. (Eds.), *Food as a drug* (pp. 123-140). New York, NY: The Haworth Press, Inc.

Haddock, C. K., & Dill, P. L. (2000). The effects of food on mood and behavior: Implications for the addictions model of obesity and eating disorders. In Poston, W. S. C. & Haddock C. K. (Eds.), *Food as a drug* (pp. 17-47). New York, NY: The Haworth Press, Inc.

Heller, R. F., & Heller, R. F. (1994). Hyperinsulinemic obesity and carbohydrate addiction: The missing link is the carbohydrate frequency. *Medical Hypotheses*, *42*, 307-312.

Howlett, M., McClelland, L., & Crisp, A. H. (1995). The cost of the illness that defies. *Postgraduate Medical Journal*, *71*, 705-711.

Hsu, L. K. (1995). Outcome of bulimia nervosa. In K. D. Brownell & C. G. Fairburn (Eds.), *Eating disorders and obesity: A comprehensive handbook* (pp. 238-244). New York: The Guilford Press.

Kirschenbaum, D. S., & Fitzgibbon, M. L. (1995). Controversy about the treatment of obesity: Criticisms or challenges? *Behavior Therapy, 26*, 43-68.

National Institutes of Health (NIH), National Heart, Lung, and Blood Institute (NHLBI). (1998). *Clinical guidelines on the identification, evaluation, and treatment of overweight and obesity: The evidence report*. U.S. Government Press: Washington D.C., 1998.

Parham, E. S. (1995). Compulsive eating: Applying a medical addiction model. In VanItallie, T. B., Simonpoulos, A. P., Gullo, S. P., & Futterweit, W. (Eds.), *Obesity: New directions in assessment and management* (pp. 185-194). Philadelphia, PA: The Charles Press.

Poston, W. S. C., Fan, L., Rakowski, R., Ericsson, M., Bunn, C. C., & Foreyt, J. P. (2000). Legal and regulatory perspectives on dietary supplements. In Poston, W. S. C. & Haddock C. K. (Eds.), *Food as a drug* (pp. 65-85). New York, NY: The Haworth Press, Inc.

Shephard, K. (1993). *Food addiction: The body knows*. Deerfield Beach, FL: Health Communications, Inc.

Stein, R. J., O'Byrne, K. K., Suminski, R. R., & Haddock, C. K. (2000). Etiology and treatment of obesity in adults and children: Implications for the addiction model. In Poston, W. S. C. & Haddock, C. K. (Eds.), *Food as a drug* (pp. 103-121). New York, NY: The Haworth Press, Inc.

Vandereycken, W., & Hoek, H. W. (1992). Are eating disorders culture-bound syndromes? In K. A. Halmi (Ed.), *Psychobiology and treatment of anorexia nervosa and bulimia nervosa* (pp. 19-36). Washington D.C.: American Psychiatric Press.

White, J. V., & Reeves, R. S. (2000). Pharmacological properties of foods and nutrients. In Poston, W. S. C. & Haddock C. K. (Eds.), *Food as a drug* (pp. 1-16). New York, NY: The Haworth Press, Inc.

Wilson, G. T. (2000). Eating Disorders and Addiction. In Poston, W. S. C. & Haddock C. K. (Eds.), *Food as a drug* (pp. 87-101). New York, NY: The Haworth Press, Inc.

World Health Organization (WHO). *Obesity: Preventing and managing the global epidemic.* Report of a WHO consultation on obesity. World Health Organization: Geneva, Switzerland, 1998.

Wurtman, J. J., & Suffes, S. (1996). *The serotonin solution: The potent substance that can help you stop bingeing, lose weight, and feel great.* New York: Fawcett Columbine.

Pharmacological Properties of Foods and Nutrients

Jane V. White, PhD, RD
Rebecca S. Reeves, DrPH, RD

SUMMARY. Nutrients, i.e., protein, carbohydrate, fat, fiber, vitamins, minerals, trace elements, and water, are commonly viewed as primary modulators of health and disease, yet they also contain many bioactive substances or "extranutritional" components. These occur naturally, are produced in vivo, or may be produced by the industrial enzymatic digestion related to various food processing activities. While these substances have been viewed as inconsequential in relation to human health, a wide range of such food constituents are recognized as having multifunctional roles in health and disease arising from the physiological, behavioral and/or immuniologic influence(s) they exert. *[Article copies available for a fee from The Haworth Document Delivery Service: 1-800-342-9678. E-mail address: getinfo@haworthpressinc.com <Website: http://www.haworthpressinc.com>]*

KEYWORDS. Macronutrients, micronutrients, bioactive substances, foods, carbohydrates

INTRODUCTION

The nutrients, i.e., protein, carbohydrate, fat, fiber, vitamins, minerals, trace elements, and water, are commonly viewed as the primary

Jane V. White is affiliated with the University of Tennessee Medical Center at Knoxville. Rebecca S. Reeves is affiliated with Baylor College of Medicine.

Address correspondence to: Jane V. White, PhD, RD, Professor, The University of Tennessee Medical Center at Knoxville, Graduate School of Medicine, Department of Family Medicine, 1924 Alcoa Highway, Knoxville, TN 37920.

[Haworth co-indexing entry note]: "Pharmacological Properties of Foods and Nutrients." White, Jane V., and Rebecca S. Reeves. Co-published simultaneously in *Drugs & Society* (The Haworth Press, Inc.) Vol. 15, No. 1/2, 1999, pp. 1-16; and: *Food as a Drug* (ed: Walker S. Carlos Poston II, and C. Keith Haddock) The Haworth Press, Inc., 2000, pp. 1-16. Single or multiple copies of this article are available for a fee from The Haworth Document Delivery Service [1-800-342-9678, 9:00 a.m. - 5:00 p.m. (EST). E-mail address: getinfo@haworthpressinc.com].

© 2000 by The Haworth Press, Inc. All rights reserved.

modulators of health and disease present in our food supply. Yet food also contains many bioactive substances or "extranutritional" components present in small quantities in the food matrix. These substances occur naturally, are produced in vivo, or may be produced by the industrial enzymatic digestion related to various food processing activities (Kitts, 1994). Although these substances have traditionally been thought to be inconsequential in relation to human health, a wide range of such food constituents are being evaluated and recognized as having multifunctional roles in health and disease arising from the physiological, behavioral and/or immuniologic influence(s) they exert.

DEFINITION OF TERMS

Specific food components are now being identified that expand the role of diet in health promotion and in the prevention and/or treatment of disease. Yet confusion abounds in this emerging area of food science-technology due to the multitude of terms that have been published in both the professional and popular press, in the United States, Europe, and Japan, in an attempt to describe and quantify advances being made in this field (Goldberg, 1994; American Dietetic Association, 1995; Bland, 1996). Table 1 lists some of the more widely used terminology and definitions.

CLASSES OF BIOACTIVE SUBSTANCES AND THEIR PURPORTED HEALTH ATTRIBUTES

The nutrients and other bioactive substances in foods are not present in isolation in a particular food item. Multiple substances capable of producing a wide array of clinical phenomena are present in each food consumed. The attribution of a particular effect or series of effects to a single food constituent is difficult, especially in the area of disease prevention/health promotion. It is more probable that the effect(s) observed results from the interplay of multiple complex substances interacting with each other and with multiple cells, organs and/or body systems in which the beneficial or harmful outcome is noted.

One way to approach this complex and confusing issue (Kitts, 1994)

TABLE 1. Definitions of Functional Foods and Related Terminology*

Term	Definition/Characteristic Elements
Chemopreventive agent	Nutritive or nonnutritive food component being scientifically investigated as a potential inhibitor of carcinogenesis for primary and secondary cancer prevention (15).
Designer food	Processed foods that are supplemented with food ingredients naturally rich in disease-preventing substances (19). This may involve genetic engineering of food.
Functional food	Any modified food or food ingredient that may provide a health benefit beyond the traditional nutrients it contains (1).
Nutraceutical	Any substance that may be considered a food or part of a food and provides medical or health benefits, including the prevention and treatment of disease (1).
Pharmafood	Food or nutrient that claims medical or health benefits, including the prevention and treatment of disease.
Phytochemical	"Substances found in edible fruits and vegetables that may be ingested by humans daily in gram quantities and that exhibit a potential for modulating human metabolism in a manner favorable for cancer prevention" (34, p. 76).

*Reprinted with permission from the American Dietetic Association Position "Phytochemicals and functional foods" (*Journal of the American Dietetic Association*, 1995; 95:493-496).

is to group bioactive substances in foods into the following broad categories based on substance origin:

- bioactive substances derived from plant products
- bioactive substances derived from animal products
- bioactive substances formed during food processing
- bioactive substances formed from the hydrolysis of food proteins

Bioactive Substances Derived from Plant Products

Glucosinolates (Thio-/Isothiocynates, Indoles, Nitrile Compounds)

Substances contained in the *Brassica* family of vegetables [broccoli, Brussels sprouts, cabbage, cauliflower, Chinese cabbage, collards, kale, kohlrabi, mustard greens, rutabaga, turnips/greens] are associated with cancer prevention in both epidemiologic and animal studies (Ensminger, 1994; Kitts, 1994). Various thiocyanates, isothiocynates, indoles, and nitrile compounds are thought to be responsible for the chemopreventive effects observed. A beneficial effect in humans has been observed for cancers of the gastrointestinal tract and genitourinary system in males and females.

Phenolic Compounds

Phenols (i.e., caffeic acid, chlorogenic acid, hydroxycinnamic acid, ferulic acid) are present in numerous foodstuffs including fruits, vegetables, tea, coffee, soybeans, and cereal grains. These substances appear to inhibit the formation of *N*-nitroso compounds thought to induce mutagenesis and carcinogenesis in humans (Kitts, 1994). Ellagic acid (grapes, strawberries, and nuts) appears to exert antineoplastic activity through stimulation of glutathione *S*-transferase activity. A phenolic component in green tea (epigallocatechin gallate) also appears to stimulate this enzyme and to exhibit antioxidant properties as well. Curcumin (curry spice, ginger), a polyphenolic compound, seems to act as both an anti-inflammatory and an antioxidant.

Flavonoids and Isoflavonoids

Flavones (i.e., luteolin, quercetin, myricetin, apigenin), found in the leaves of cereal crops and isoflavones (i.e., genistein, formononetin, diadzeim), are found in lentils, soybeans, licorice root and flax seed. These compounds appear to have strong antioxidative properties as evidenced by the chelation of metals or by free radical scavenging. Their purported antitumor and lipid lowering effects appear to be linked to inhibition of cyclooxygenase and lipoxygenase activity. Some of the isoflavonoids exhibit weak estrogenic/antiestrogenic activity and are termed phytoestrogens, substances thought to be important in the prevention of lipid disorders and certain cancers (Kitts, 1994).

Terpenes

Essential oils (terpenes) from numerous plant sources including caraway seeds, dill weed, oranges, grapefruit, lemon, spearmint, and green coffee beans have been shown to have anticarcinogenic and lipid lowering properties in animals and humans (Kitts, 1994).

Organosulfur Compounds

Anticarcinogenic, antimutagenic, and lipid lowering activity have been reported for compounds contained within the group of plants of the genus *Allium* (chives, garlic, leeks, onion, shallot) (Sorrentino,

1998; Berthold, 1998). The allyl di- and trisulfides present in these plants appear to stimulate glutathione peroxidase and glutathione *S*-transferase and to inhibit glutathione reductase, acetyl CoA synthetase and ornithine decarboxylase activities.

Other Plant Constituents

Alpha-tocotrienol in barley, coumarins and phthalides in umbelliferous vegetables and herbs (i.e., anise, caraway, carrot, celery, coriander, cumin, dill, fennel, parsley, parsnip, rutabaga), and quinones in rosemary exhibit anticarcinogenic and antioxidant activity similar to synthetic antioxidants such as butylated hydroxyanisol (BHA) and butylated hydroxytolulene (BHT).

Bioactive Substances Derived from Animal Products

There appear to be both mutagenic and tumor-modulating substances produced during the microsomal enzymatic degradation of protein and fats in meat and diary products (Kitts, 1994). An example is C-9,C-12 octadecadienoic acid (CLA), a derivative of linolenic acid found in heat-processed meats and dairy products that displays both antioxidant and anticarcinogenic properties.

In addition, a number of bioactive peptides are present naturally in foods (i.e., growth co-factors in milk) that produce both direct effects on the availability of nutrients and indirect effects on peripheral organs (Kitts, 1994; Goldberg, 1994). Peptides derived from the digestion of casein are associated with a number of biological effects including antihypertensive activity, opioid inhibition or stimulation, immunomodulation, and antithrombotic effects. Casein phosphopeptides also function as carriers for different minerals, especially calcium (Meisel, 1997).

The curing of meat yields both nitrosoamines, implicated in mutagenesis and carcinogenesis, and nitrosylhaem pigments which act as free radical scavengers and protect both the meat pigment and the lipids contained in the meat from oxidation (Eriksson, 1995). The true physiologic significance of bioactive peptides derived from foods is poorly understood.

Bioactive Substances Formed During Food Processing

The majority of foods consumed in the United States undergoes some form of processing (physical or chemical operation applied to a foodstuff) before reaching the table (Ensminger, 1994). These actions tend to enhance the level of certain nutrients while reducing the levels of others. Many commonly used processing methods tend to concentrate solids, carbohydrates, fats, and/or proteins at the expense of fiber, certain essential vitamins and/or minerals. The risk-benefit ratios of highly processed foods must be carefully considered because they have the potential to meet specific, even highly specialized nutrient needs while providing pitfalls that must be recognized and addressed.

Heating foods (i.e., baking, roasting, broiling, frying) or prolonged food storage causes aminocarbonyl reactions which alter food acceptance by changing its color, odor, and/or taste (Ensminger, 1994). Maillard reaction (nonenzymatic browning caused by reactions between sugars and amino acids) products (MRPs) display both mutagenic and antimutagenic activity depending on the reaction substrates. Some protein-polysaccharide conjugates increase the emulsifying activity, as well as the antioxidative and antimicrobial effects of the original proteins (Chuyen, 1998). Some types of heat treatment induce the formation of new compounds with antioxidant effects such as the formation of MRPs. Thermal treatment of tomatoes and coffee, although significantly reducing the concentration of naturally occurring antioxidants in these foodstuffs, resulted in the development of MRPs which significantly enhanced the overall antioxidant properties of these items (Nicoli, 1997; Sites, 1998).

Polycyclic aromatic hydrocarbons (PAH) in processed foods are caused by certain food preservation and processing procedures. Both toxicologic and epidemiologic studies have shown a relation between these compounds and tumor development (Guillen, 1997). Food processing and packaging procedures should be modified to ensure that PAH contamination is kept to a minimum.

Trans fatty acids, produced during the hydrogenation of oils and used as saturated fat replacements in foods and food processing, are thought to be highly atherogenic. Compared to the saturated fatty acids it was designed to replace, elaidic acid [dietary trans 18:1] significantly elevated total LDL cholesterol and uniquely depressed HDL cholesterol in male and female subjects consuming moderate-to-low fat, low cholesterol whole food diets. Its negative effect on serum lipids was unmatched by any other natural fatty acid studied (Sundrum, 1997).

Bioactive Substances Formed from the Hydrolysis of Food Proteins

The addition of enzymes to food, while offering considerable potential for food improvement, also offers considerable potential for rapid deterioration of food quality when used indiscriminately or in poorly controlled circumstances (James, 1996; Ashie, 1996). Although any of the major biomolecules found in foods can be manipulated through enzyme addition, this process has most consistently been applied to food proteins. Some proteins arising from the enzymatic hydrolysis of casein, gluten, and fish protein have considerable biologic activity.

Protein hydrolysates (peptones) from egg albumin and meat appear to control the secretion and/or the synthesis of gut hormones (Cordier-Bussat, 1998; Nemoz-Gaillard, 1998). Angiotensin I-converting enzyme (ACE) inhibitory peptides have been recovered from the protein hydrolysis of a number of food system proteins including casein and fish and are associated with reductions of systolic blood pressure in animal models. Depending on the enzyme used and the peptide bond hydrolyzed, potency and resistance to further peptide hydrolysis can be achieved (Yokoyama, 1992). Peptides derived from the digestion of cereal and milk proteins (β-casomorphins) seem to exhibit opioid activity and thus may affect appetite, behavior and intestinal motility in selected individuals (Kitts, 1994).

BIOACTIVE SUBSTANCES IN FOOD AND MOOD

A number of issues must be considered when evaluating the impact of foods/food components on mood. Inconsistencies in assessment of the impact of individual variation on study outcome and lack of standardization regarding the degree of food/food component use, presence of psychological or psychiatric disorders, and the type of test used to measure mood/attitude and/or various aspects of function (sensory, physical, cognitive) make consensus regarding study outcomes difficult. Reliable, integrated measures to assess food's impact on function (i.e., overall job performance) are lacking (Goldberg, 1994). Below is a brief review of the scientific literature regarding this issue.

Calories (Energy)

During the last 10-15 years, research has demonstrated that women consume significantly more calories during the premenstrual (luteal) phase of their cycle than at other times during the month (Kurzer, 1997). Caloric consumption in healthy women increases in the range of 90-500 kcal per day. Similar findings have been observed in women with premenstrual syndrome (PMS). Increases in carbohydrate, protein, and fat intakes have all been reported, as has increased consumption of vitamin D, riboflavin, potassium, phosphorus and magnesium. Causes of increased premenstrual food intake in women are unknown. Despite numerous studies and claims to the contrary, consistent food cravings or preferences have not been identified.

A number of studies have looked at the effect of food consumption on the performance of mental tasks and the subjective feelings of mood. A number of variables other than the specific food components fed influence study outcomes including the timing of the meal, nutritional status of the subjects being fed, habitual patterns of food intake, beliefs about food and the nature of the mental tasks to be performed. In a recent review, Kanarek (1997) concluded that breakfast intake is generally associated with an improvement in cognitive performance later in the morning, while lunch intake is associated with impaired mid-afternoon performance of mental tasks and more negative mood reports. Intake of food late in the afternoon appears to enhance performance of tasks requiring sustained attention or memory. No definitive conclusions regarding meal composition or food components could be drawn.

Caloric consumption appears to affect pain perception in both males and females (Zmarzty, 1997). A cold pressor test was administered before and after subjects were fed a high-fat low-carbohydrate meal, high-carbohydrate low-fat meal, or no meal. Mean pain scores were significantly reduced following the consumption of both meals versus when no food was consumed. The greatest reduction in pain scores was observed at 1.5 hours post ingestion of the high-fat meal.

Fats and Cholesterol

A study by Wells and Read (1996) in 18 male subjects suggests that in the early morning, fat consumption tends to depress alertness and mood to a greater extent than does carbohydrate ingestion irrespective of the energy content of the meal fed. This effect tends to diminish as the day progresses and is less evident at lunch time. A companion study (Wells, Read, Uvnas-Moberg, & Alster, 1997) suggested an association between the lassitude experienced after a meal and release of cholecystokinin (CCK). Ratings of fatigue in these subjects were greatest 3 hours after consumption of a high-fat low-carbohydrate meal.

When fed isocaloric lunches differing in fat and carbohydrate content, subjects rated themselves as more drowsy, uncertain, muddled, and less cheerful when consuming low-fat high-carbohydrate or high-fat low-carbohydrate lunches than when consuming moderate-fat moderate-carbohydrate meals (Lloyd, 1994). They reported feeling less tense after the low-fat high-carbohydrate meal. It would appear that higher than usual proportions of both fat and carbohydrate produce a relative impairment of cognitive efficiency.

Wells, Read, Laugharne, and Ahluwalia (1998) showed that a reduction in dietary fat content from 41% to 25% of total calories significantly increased profile of mood states ratings of anger-hostility in subjects consuming the low fat diet even though no changes in serum cholesterol, LDL-cholesterol and triglyceride levels were observed. However, the duration of this study was one month and serum cholesterol values don't necessarily respond to diet or drug interventions in this short a span of time. Fries et al. (1997) reported that subjects experienced stronger negative emotions when they were simply told that their usual diet was high in fat. However, these subjects capitalized on the negative emotions experienced when this information was provided by expressing stronger intentions to lower fat intake than subjects who were told that their usual food intakes were low or moderate in fat.

Epidemiological and experimental data (Kaplan, 1997) also suggest that naturally low or diet/drug induced reductions in serum cholesterol are associated with increased incidence of suicide and accidents. It is hypothesized that alterations in dietary or plasma cholesterol adversely impact mood and that such effects are potentiated by lipid-induced changes in brain chemistry possibly through a mechanism involving central serotonergic activity. Further studies in this area are needed.

Carbohydrate

Wurtman and Wurtman (1995) suggested that carbohydrate consumption–acting via insulin secretion and the "plasma tryptophan ratio"–increases serotonin release while keeping protein and carbohydrate intakes relatively constant. However, because serotonin release is also associated with sleep onset, pain sensitivity, blood pressure regulation and mood control, many people learn to overeat carbohydrate dense snacks (which also tend to be high in fat) to make themselves feel better. A number of recent studies suggest limited agreement with this theory.

In women suffering from PMS (Sayegh, 1995), consumption of a specially formulated carbohydrate-rich beverage (designed to increase serum tryptophan levels) decreased self-reported depression, anger, confusion, and carbohydrate craving 90-180 minutes after ingestion. Memory word recognition also improved significantly. Placebo beverage consumption had no significant impact on any of the measures assessed.

Markus et al. (1998) showed that when individuals who were highly stress-prone were subjected to an uncontrollable stress situation, those consuming a carbohydrate-rich protein-poor diet were able to increase personal control and avoided the negative effects on pulse rate, skin conductance, cortisol levels and mood experienced by those consuming the protein-rich carbohydrate-poor diet.

Paz and Berry (1997) looked at the effect of diet composition on performance during and after self selected night-shift work. They compared subjective alertness, psychometric performance, and plasma levels of insulin, glucose and amino acids (tyrosine:tryptophan ratio) when subjects were fed 3 diets: one high protein (52%), one high carbohydrate (70%), or the workers' regular diet (18% protein, 55% carbohydrate). The fat content of the diets was held constant at 27%. The regular diet gave the best performance; insulin and glucose levels were similar among diets. The authors suggest that a carbohydrate:protein ratio of 3 may result in optimal balance between mood and performance during night-shift work.

Due to the preponderance of low fat, high carbohydrate (sucrose) foods present in today's marketplace, Surwit et al. (1997) examined the impact of high versus low sucrose, low fat hypocaloric diets on a number of behavioral and metabolic indices over a 6 week period. Diet composition was 11% fat, 19% protein, and 71% carbohydrate with the diet high in sucrose containing 43% of total calories as sucrose and the low sucrose diet containing 4% total calories as sucrose. The impact of both diets on weight loss, blood pressure, resting energy expenditure and plasma lipids was similar; both groups showed decreases in hunger, depression, and negative mood and increases in vigilance and positive mood over time.

Amino Acids

In normal weight women who have bulimia nervosa, it is postulated that serotonin activity is reduced. To examine this hypothesis, Weltzin et al. (1995) examined the effect of acute tryptophan depletion in 10 women with bulimia and in 10 normal controls. The women with bulimia showed an increase in caloric intake and mood irritability following acute tryptophan depletion. Other studies suggest that dysregulation of serotonergic pathways in the central nervous system may contribute to core symptoms in patients with eating disorders (Wolfe, 1997; Verri, 1997).

Earlier studies have suggested roles for tyrosine and phenylalanine in addition to tryptophan in the regulation of brain neurotransmission. The impact of administration of these protein components on behavior remains controversial (Goldman, 1994).

Chocolate

Food cravings are experienced by approximately 68% of men and 97% of women. The most frequently reported food craving among college aged women is for chocolate (Hill, 1994; Kurzer, 1997). Between 39-49% of all food cravings in women are for this substance. In men, the craving for chocolate is experienced by approximately 14%, about the same percentage that experience a craving for pizza. Although numerous theories have been proposed to explain women's craving for chocolate and for food cravings in general, little consensus has been reached. Chocolate does contain a number of bioactive substances including methylxanthines (theobromine, caffeine), neurotransmitter precursors (phenylalanine, tyrosine), biogenoic amines (phenylethylamine, tyramine) and magnesium. However, when subjects were fed substances which contained the components of chocolate without its flavor, sweetness, or recognizable form, the craving for chocolate remained unsatisfied (Michener, 1994). These findings would seem to suggest that the craving for chocolate is due to its sensory or psychologic attributes rather than to its pharmacologic effects. The findings of Macdiarmid and Heatherington (1995) tend to support this contention.

Caffeine/Coffee

Coffee (containing the methylxanthine caffeine) is used to improve mood by many people. A 10-year study by Kawachi et al. (1996)

examined the relationship of coffee and caffeine intake to risk of suicide in women. A strong inverse relationship was found between coffee intake and caffeine intake from all sources and risk of suicide. Compared with non-drinkers of coffee, the age adjusted relative risk of suicide in women who drank 2-3 cups per day was 0.34 [CI 0.17-0.68] and for women who consumed 4 or more cups per day 0.42 [CI 0.21 to 0.86]. These findings were unchanged after adjusting for a wide range of factors.

Quinlan (1997) assessed the temporal effects on psychological and physiologic function that caffeine, hot water, or beverage type has on observed effects of beverage consumption. The addition of milk and 100 mg of caffeine also was assessed. The impact of sugar addition was not assessed. Heating beverages rapidly increased skin conductance and temperature. This effect was observed 10-30 minutes post ingestion. Caffeine in the beverage reduced skin temperature response but increased both systolic and diastolic blood pressure 30-60 minutes post consumption. Both caffeine and milk addition to beverages independently improved mood and reduced anxiety 30-60 minutes post consumption. Responses to tea and coffee consumption were similar but tea potentiated the increase in skin temperature compared to coffee and water possibly due to the presence of flavonoids in tea. Beverage temperature, type, and milk addition play an important modulary role in responses to caffeine ingestion.

Opioids

The impact of opioids (produced in response to food or present in foods) on appetite was assessed in subjects consuming pasta with either cheese or tomato sauce (Yeomans, 1997). When naltrexone (an opiate antagonist) was administered prior to eating, subjects ate significantly less of both foods. Pleasantness ratings for food and overall eating rate were also reduced. Although naltrexone seemed to exert a mild sedative effect in subjects, changes in alertness alone could not account for naltrexone's impact on appetite. It was suggested that opioids stimulate appetite through an effect on food palatability.

Chicken Extract

Folklore has it that chicken soup is useful in the recovery from physical and mental distress. Nagai (1996) tested this assumption by assessing the effectiveness of chicken extract (BEC) on the recovery from mental stress by examining blood levels of cortisol, task performance, and mood during mental task (simple math and short term memory assessment) performance. Male subjects who consumed BEC had shorter mean cortisol level recovery times and better task performance compared to those receiving a placebo. Subjects felt more active and less fatigued during the workload when BEC was regularly consumed.

Vitamin D

Seasonal mood changes are reported to affect some individuals with anxiety and depression which increase as winter progresses. Seasonal affective disorder is associated with carbohydrate craving, hypersomnia, lethargy, and changes in circadian rhythm. Some have postulated that these mood disturbances may be linked to changes in circulating levels of Vitamin D3, the hormone produced by sun exposure. Reduced levels of circulating Vitamin D3 are postulated to lead to changes in brain serotonin. When healthy subjects were given varying doses or no Vitamin D3 for 5 days during late winter, results of a self-report showed that Vitamin D3 significantly enhanced positive affect and reduced negative affect (Lansdowne, 1998). The seasonal variation observed in serum Vitamin D3 levels does not affect serum levels of 1,25-dihydroxy-vitamin D (Hine, 1994).

Vitamin C

Substitution of the sensory cues of smoking with a citric acid aerosol significantly reduces craving for cigarettes and enhances smoking reduction and cessation in people trying to quit smoking cigarettes (Levin, 1993). A cigarette-sized tube which delivered a fine aerosol of ascorbic acid (1 mg/puff up to a maximum of 300 mg/day) was used in this trial. The group using the device showed significantly greater abstinence rates at 3 weeks post cigarette cessation. After subjects stopped using the device, no difference in abstinence was detected. Negative mood was also lower in subjects receiving ascorbate. The mechanism of action of this effect is not known although smokers' requirement for vitamin C is greater than that of non-smokers.

CONCLUSION

The impact of food, nutrients and bioactive substances in food on mood and behavior has yet to be elucidated. The most prudent advice that can be offered at this time is consumption of a varied diet, rich in grains, fruit, vegetables and low fat dairy products and moderate in animal protein, alcohol, and fat, so that a nutritionally adequate intake is assured.

REFERENCES

American Dietetic Association. (1995). Position of the American Dietetic Association: Phytochemicals and functional foods. *Journal of the American Dietetic Association, 95*, 493-496.

Ashie, I. N., Simpson, B. K., and Smith, J. P. (1996). Mechanisms for controlling enzymatic reactions in foods. *Critical Reviews in Food Science and Nutrition, 36*, 1-30.

Bland, J. S. (1996). Phytonutrition, phytotherapy, and phytopharmacology. *Alternative Therapies in Health and Medicine, 2(6)*, 73-76.

Berthold, H. K., Sudhop, T., and von Bergmann, K. (1998). Effect of a garlic oil preparation on serum lipoproteins and cholesterol metabolism. *JAMA, 279*, 1900-1902.

Chuyen, N. V. (1998). Maillard reaction and food processing. application aspects. *Advances in Experimental Medicine and Biology, 434*, 213-235.

Cordier-Bussat, M., Bernard, C., Levenez, F., Klages, N., Laser-Ritz, B., Philippe, J., Chayvialle, J. A., and Cuber, J. (1998). Peptones stimulate both the secretion of the incretin hormone glucagon-like peptide and the transcription of the proglucagon gene. *Diabetes, 47*, 1038-1045.

Ensminger, A. H., Ensminger, M. E., Konlande, J. E., and Robson, J. R. K. (1994). *Foods & Nutrition Encyclopedia*. Bocca Raton, FL: CRC Press.

Eriksson, C. E., and Na, A. (1995). Antioxidant agents in raw materials and processed foods. *Biochemical Society Symposia, 61*, 221-234.

Fries, E. A., Bowen, D. J., Hopp, H. P., and White, K. S. (1997). Psychological effects of dietary fat analysis and feedback: A randomized feedback design. *Journal of Behavioral Medicine, 20*, 607-619.

Goldberg, I. (1994). *Functional Foods: Designer Foods, Pharmafoods, Nutraceuticals*. New York, NY: Chapman & Hall.

Guillen, M. D., Sopelana, P., and Partearroyo, M. A. (1997). Food as a source of polycyclic aromatic carcinogens. *Reviews of Environmental Health, 12*, 133-146.

Hill, A. J., and Heaton-Brown, L. (1994). The experience of food craving: A prospective investigation in healthy women. *Journal of Psychosomatic Research, 38*, 801-814.

Hine, T. J., and Roberts, N. B. (1994). Seasonal variation in serum 25-hydroxy vitamin D3 does not affect 1,25-dihydroxy vitamin D. *Annals of Clinical Biochemistry, 31(pt 1)*, 31-34.

James, J., and Simpson, B. K. (1996). Application of enzymes in food processing. *Crit Reviews of Food Science and Nutrition, 36*, 437-463.

Kanarek, R. (1997). Psychological effects of snacks and altered meal frequency. *British Journal of Nutrition, 77 Suppl 1*, 118-20.

Kaplan, J. R., Muldoon, M. F., Manuck, S. B., and Mann, J. J. (1997). Assessing the observed relationship between low cholesterol and violence-related mortality. Implications for suicide risk. *Annals of the New York Academy of Science, 836*, 57-80.

Kawachi, I., Willett, W. C., Colditz, G. A., Stampfer, M. J., and Speizer. F. E. (1996). A prospective study of coffee drinking and suicide. *Archives of Internal Medicine, 156*, 521-525.

Kitts, D. D. (1994). Bioactive substances in food: Identification and potential uses. *Canadian Journal of Physiology and Pharmacology,72*, 423-434.

Kurzer, M. S. (1997). Women, food, and mood. *Nutrition Reviews, 55*, 268-276.

Lansdowne, A. T., and Provost, S. C. (1998). Vitamin D3 enhances mood in healthy subjects during winter. *Psychopharmacology, 135*, 319-323.

Lloyd, H. M., Green, M. W., and Rogers, P. J. (1994). Mood and cognitive performance effects of isocaloric lunches differing in fat and carbohydrate content. *Physiology and Behavior, 56*, 51-57.

Macdiarmid, J. I., and Hetherington, M. M. (1995). Mood modulation by food: An exploration of affect and cravings in 'chocolate addicts.' *British Journal of Clinical Psychology, 34(Pt 1)*, 129-138.

Markus, C. R., Panhuysen, G., Tuiten, A., Koppeschaar, H., Fekkes, D., and Peters, M. L. (1998). Does carbohydrate-rich, protein-poor food prevent a deterioration of mood and cognitive performance of stress-prone subjects when subjected to a stressful task? *Appetite, 31*, 49-65.

Meisel, H. (1997). Biochemical properties of regulatory peptides derived from milk proteins. *Biopolymers, 43*, 119-128.

Michner, W., and Rozin, P. (1994). Pharmacological versus sensory factors in the satiation of chocolate craving. *Physiology and Behavior, 56*, 419-422.

Nagai, H., Harada, M., Nakagawa, M., Tanaka, T., Gunadi, B., Setiabudi, M. L., Uktolseja, J. L., and Miyata, Y. (1996). Effects of chicken extract on the recovery from fatigue caused by mental workload. *Applied Human Science, 15*, 281-286.

Nemoz-Gaillard, E., Bernard, C., Abello, J., Cordier-Bussat, M., Chayvialle, J. A., and Cuber, J. C. (1998). Regulation of cholecystokinin secretion by peptides and peptidomimetic antibiotics in SCT-1 cells. *Endocrinology, 139*, 932-938.

Nicoli, M. C., Anese, M., Parpinel, M. T., Franceschi, S., and Lerici, C. R. (1997). Loss and/or formation of antioxidants during food processing and storage. *Cancer Letters, 114(1-2)*, 71-74.

Paz, A., and Berry, E. M. (1997). Effect of meal composition on alertness and performance of hospital night-shift workers. Do mood and performance have different determinants? *Annals of Nutrition and Metabolism, 41*, 291-298.

Quinlan, P., Lane, J., and Aspinall, L. (1997). Effects of hot tea, coffee and water ingestion on physiological responses and mood: The role of caffeine, water and beverage type. *Psychopharmacology, 134*, 164-73.

Sayegh, R., Schiff, I., Wurtman, J., Spiers, P., McDermott, J., and Wurtman, R.

(1995). The effect of a carbohydrate-rich beverage on mood, appetite, and cognitive function in women with premenstrual syndrome. *Obstetrics and Gynecology, 86(4 Pt 1),* 520-528.

Sies, H., and Stahl, W. (1998). Lycopene: Antioxidant and biological effects and its bioavailability in the human. *Proceedings of the Society for Experimental Biology and Medicine, 218,* 121-124.

Sorrentino, M. (1998). Garlic: Is the "stinking rose" good for the cholesterol count? *Alternative Medicine Alert., 1,* 97-99.

Sundram, K., Ismail, A., Hayes, K. C., Jeyamalar, R., and Pathmanathan, R. (1997). Trans (elaidic) fatty acids adversely affect the lipoprotein profile relative to specific saturated fatty acids in humans. *Journal of Nutrition, 127,* 514S-520S.

Surwit, R. S., Feinglos, M. N., McCaskill, C. C., Clay, S. L., Babyak, M. A., Brownlow, B. S., Plaisted, C. S., and Lin, P. H. (1997). Metabolic and behavioral effects of a high-sucrose diet during weight loss. *American Journal of Clinical Nutrition, 65,* 908-915.

Verri, A., Nappi, R. E., Vallero, E., Galli, C., Sances, G., and Martignoni, E. (1997). Premenstrual dysphoric disorder and eating disorders. *Cephalalgia, 17 suppl 20,* 25-28.

Wells, A. S., and Read, N. W. (1996). Influences of fat, energy, and time of day on mood and performance. *Physiology and Behavior, 59,* 1069-1076.

Wells, A. S., Read, N. W., Laugharne, J. D., and Ahluwalia, N. S. (1998). Alterations in mood after changing to a low fat diet. *British Journal of Nutrition, 79,* 23-30.

Wells, A. S., Read, N. W., Uvnas-Moberg, K., and Alster, P. (1997). Influences of fat and carbohydrate on postprandial sleepiness, mood, and hormones. *Physiolology and Behavior, 61,* 679-686.

Wolfe, B. E., Metzger, E., and Jimerson, D. C. (1997). Research update on serotonin function in bulimia nervosa and anorexia nervosa. *Psychopharmacology Bulletin, 33,* 345-354.

Wurtman, R. J., and Wurtman, J. J. (1995). Brain serotonin, carbohydrate-craving, obesity and depression. *Obesity Research, 3 Suppl 4,* 477S-480S.

Yokoyama, K., Chiba, H., and Yoshikawa, M. (1992). Peptide inhibition for angiotensin I-converting enzyme from thermolysin digest of dried bonito. *Bioscience, Biotechnology, and Biochemistry, 50,* 2419-2421.

Yomans, M. R., and Gray, R. W. (1997). Effects of naltrexone on food intake and changes in subjective appetite during eating: Evidence for opioid involvement in the appetizer effect. *Physiology and Behavior, 62,* 15-21.

Zmarzty, S. A., Wells, A. S., and Read, N. W. (1997). The influence of food on pain perception in healthy human volunteers. *Physiology and Behavior, 62,* 185-191.

The Effects of Food on Mood and Behavior: Implications for the Addictions Model of Obesity and Eating Disorders

C. Keith Haddock, PhD
Patricia L. Dill, MS

SUMMARY. The addictions model of obesity claims that individuals gain excess weight due to their dependence on and inability to control the intake of certain food substances. The dependence and lack of control over these food substances is undergirded by, according to the addictions model, the psychoactive properties of foods. The article reviews the literature on the purported psychoactive effects of foods and concludes that although, under certain circumstances, some food substances may have subtle effects on mood and behavior, the effects of food are quite different from that of psychoactive drugs such as nicotine and alcohol. Therefore, the food addictions model is unlikely to provide a fruitful paradigm for understanding the complex problem of obesity. *[Article copies available for a fee from The Haworth Document Delivery Service: 1-800-342-9678. E-mail address: getinfo@haworthpressinc.com <Website: http://www.haworth pressinc.com>]*

C. Keith Haddock is Assistant Professor, Department of Psychology, University of Missouri-Kansas City and Co-Director of Behavioral Cardiology Research, Mid America Heart Institute, St. Luke's Hospital. Patricia L. Dill is affiliated with the University of Missouri-Kansas City.

Address correspondence to: C. Keith Haddock, PhD, Department of Psychology, University of Missouri-Kansas City, 5319 Holmes, Kansas City, MO 64110 (E-mail: haddockc@umkc.edu).

The authors would like to thank Dr. Kathy Goggin, Dr. Charles Sheridan, and Dr. Risa J. Stein for their comments on initial drafts of this manuscript. However, the content, including its shortcomings, is the responsibility of the authors.

This article was supported by a Faculty Research Grant awarded to Dr. Haddock by the University of Missouri-Kansas City.

[Haworth co-indexing entry note]: "The Effects of Food on Mood and Behavior: Implications for the Addictions Model of Obesity and Eating Disorders." Haddock, C. Keith, and Patricia L. Dill. Co-published simultaneously in *Drugs & Society* (The Haworth Press, Inc.) Vol. 15, No. 1/2, 1999, pp. 17-47; and: *Food as a Drug* (ed: Walker S. Carlos Poston II, and C. Keith Haddock) The Haworth Press, Inc., 2000, pp. 17-47. Single or multiple copies of this article are available for a fee from The Haworth Document Delivery Service [1-800-342-9678, 9:00 a.m. - 5:00 p.m. (EST). E-mail address: getinfo@haworthpressinc.com].

© 2000 by The Haworth Press, Inc. All rights reserved.

KEYWORDS. Pharmacological, carbohydrates, sugar, mood, addiction, diet, depression, hyperactivity

Throughout history, claims that certain foods act as powerful drugs are commonplace (Christensen, 1996). Individuals have been warned to avoid various foods because of their adverse effects while specific diets are offered as cures to common diseases and psychological problems. Combined with the fact that many overweight individuals appear to eat in a compulsive manner, many in the popular press (Minirth, 1991; Sheppard, 1993) and in professional journals (e.g., Kayloe, 1993; Yeary, 1987) have suggested that obesity is due to a drug dependence disorder similar to that found for alcohol or nicotine. That is, the obese individual is a "food addict" who has become pharmacologically dependent on certain food substances.

Within the addictions model of obesity, food addiction is defined as obsession with food, obsession with weight, and loss of control over the amount of food eaten, and the compulsive pursuit of a mood change by engaging in episodes of binge eating despite adverse consequences (Sheppard, 1993; Kayloe, 1993). The etiology of food addiction is said to lie in a physiological, biochemical condition of the body that creates cravings for refined carbohydrates and other food substances (Sheppard, 1993). Furthermore, as with other drug dependencies, Sheppard (1993) suggests that a genetic susceptibility separates a person who may develop a food addiction from other individuals. Assuming that the obese individual's craving for food is comparable to the alcoholic's craving for alcohol, Sheppard (1993) notes that the proper therapeutic regimen for food addiction involves abstinence from highly refined carbohydrate foods, foods high in fat, and the individual's personal trigger foods. These sentiments are illustrated in the following quotes from a popular book on food addiction (Sheppard, 1989):

> Can gummy bears and marshmallow chicks really be vicious killers? As silly as that sounds, the truth of the matter is that for certain individuals who are sensitive, refined carbohydrates can trigger the addictive process. (p. xi)

> Food addiction is not less than any other addiction in terms of suffering and adverse consequences. It can be a fatal error for

food addicts to minimize the serious nature of this disease. Our morgues and hospitals are filled with its victims. (p. xii)

The addictions model of obesity is the treatment philosophy of one of the largest self-help organizations for the obese in the United States–Overeaters Anonymous (OA). The first OA meeting was held on January 19, 1960, and since that time this approach to treatment has garnered increasing popularity (Yeary, 1987). Although a recent OA member survey suggests that involvement has decreased markedly over the past decade (OA, 1997-1998), the organization claims that between 41,516 and 83,052 individuals currently participate in OA meetings. Modeled after Alcoholics Anonymous (AA), the OA philosophy states that food and weight problems are not due to a lack of willpower or a moral defect, but are the result of a disease that can be arrested. OA subscribes to a 12-step, disease model of treatment. The 12-steps of OA include the assertions that the individual is powerless over food and that they must rely on a higher power in order to control their addiction to food substances.

Is obesity appropriately characterized as the result of a drug dependence similar to that found for alcohol and nicotine? The answer to this question depends on how closely one requires the dietary behaviors of the obese to match accepted criteria for drug dependence (see Table 1). The primary criteria of drug dependence are (1) highly controlled or compulsive use, (2) the substance used is mood-altering or psychoactive effects are central elements of the drug's activity, and (3) the drug has the demonstrated capability of reinforcing behavior (USDHHS, 1988; 1994). Other important diagnostic criteria include tolerance and physical dependence. Whether the eating style of the obese can be characterized along any of the criteria used for establishing drug dependence has been seriously challenged (e.g., Parham, 1995; Vandereycken, 1990; Wilson, 1991; 1999). For instance, Vandereycken (1990) suggests that attributing obesity and other eating disorders to food addiction is a case of "reasoning by analogy" and posits that "this much too common habit in psychiatry and psychology has two major pitfalls: (1) *selective reduction,* i.e., according to some facets of the overeating behavior and its concomitant cognitions and emotions, specific resemblances are stressed but differences are minimized or ignored; and (2) *overgeneralization,* i.e., the identification of

various forms of overeating as being variants of one core-behavior"
(p. 96).

Although many behaviors are habitual and difficult to control,
drug addictions are unique due to the psychoactive properties of the
abused substance (USDHHS; 1994). That is, the addict becomes
dependent on the mood or behavior altering effects of the drug.
Therefore, a key piece of evidence needed to establish obesity as a
drug dependence disorder involves demonstrating that foods within
the obese individual's diet have psychoactive properties that significantly alter mood and behavior. Not surprisingly, advocates of the
addictions model of obesity view food as a powerful psychoactive
substance. For instance, Yeary (1987, p. 305) writes, "One way to
view eating disorders is to appreciate that food is a complex mixture
of chemicals and that the body responds to food as it does to chemicals, such as those found in alcohol and other psychoactive drugs.
Eating disorders are therefore chemical disorders." Thus, the purpose of this article is to review the evidence regarding whether dietary substances can significantly alter mood and behavior in a manner similar to psychoactive drugs.

TABLE 1. Criteria for Drug Dependence

---

(1) Primary Criteria

    Highly controlled or compulsive behavior

    Psychoactive effects

    Drug-reinforced behavior

(2) Additional Criteria

  Addictive behavior often involves the following:

    Stereotypic pattern of use

    Use despite harmful effects

    Relapse following abstinence

    Recurrent drug cravings

  Dependence-producing drugs often manifest the following:

    Tolerance

    Physical dependence

    Pleasant (euphoric) effects

Source: USDHHS 1988; 1994

THE PSYCHOACTIVE EFFECTS OF FOOD

Sugar and certain food additives cause Attention Deficit Hyperactivity Disorder. Hypoglycemia, caused by high sucrose consumption, leads to juvenile delinquency. Although many readers will quickly dismiss such claims as unsupported and simplistic, these assertions were once supported by serious researchers and appeared in peer-review publications in the scientific literature (Christensen, 1996). The literature is replete with examples of initial enthusiasm regarding the effect of food substances on mood and behavior followed by failures to replicate and, ultimately, rejection of the notion that the food substances have important psychoactive characteristics. As a result, the scientific community is generally skeptical of suggestions that foods significantly alter mood or behavior (Spring, Chiodo, & Bowen, 1987). In fact, in the revision of the third edition of the *Diagnostic and Statistical Manual of Mental Disorders* (*DSM-IIIR*), (American Psychiatric Association [APA], 1987) there was an attempt to exclude food from consideration as an addictive substance by using the term "psychoactive substance" rather than the general term "substance" when addressing addictive disorders (Rounsaville, Spitzer, & Williams, 1986). Apparently, the authors of the *DSM-IIIR* did not consider foods to be psychoactive drugs.

Is the skepticism among scientists regarding the purported psychoactive effects of food justified? There is substantial evidence that deficiencies in certain vitamins can lead to profound changes in mood and behavior (Christensen, 1996). However, the psychoactive effects of undereating are generally not presented as an important factor in the food addictions model of obesity and significant nutrition deficiencies are not common among the obese (Parham, 1995). In terms of whole foods normally eaten, it is unlikely that the consumption of any widely available food substances will dramatically affect mood or behavior. Lieberman and colleagues (Lieberman, Spring, & Garfield, 1986) note that food constituents (with the possible exception of caffeine) do not interact directly with synaptic macromolecules or accumulate in vivo. Therefore, any effects on mood or behavior are likely to be subtle and hard to detect. Even when various food substances are administered in large quantities and in pure form, they demonstrate little pharmacological effect (Lieberman et al., 1986; Neims, 1986). Therefore, most scientists have concluded that food cannot be considered truly psychoactive (Parham, 1996), a fact which seriously challenges the validity of the food addictions model of obesity (Wilson, 1991; 1999).

If most serious scientists have concluded that foods are not truly psychoactive, then why is the food addictions model of obesity widely accepted by many in the general public? In the remainder of this article we will examine the rise and fall of what once was a widely accepted relationship between diet and behavior in children. We will examine how anecdotal reports and flawed studies lead to the widespread belief that sugar and certain food additives can lead to hyperactivity and aggression in children. Furthermore, we will show that despite the emergence of strong evidence to the contrary, the belief that diet is responsible for hyperactivity remains influential in the general public. Finally, we will conclude with an overview of a food-mood relationship with strong empirical support–the effect of dietary tryptophan on depression. Although there is an established connection between tryptophan and mood, the effects of dietary tryptophan are subtle and only occur under highly prescribed circumstances. We will also examine the proposition that one group of obese individuals are particularly responsive to the effects of tryptophan on mood–those with a strong preference for carbohydrate-rich foods or "carbohydrate cravers."

IS HYPERACTIVITY CAUSED BY THE PSYCHOACTIVE PROPERTIES OF DIET?

The notion that certain foods had a negative effect on the behavior of children dates from at least 1922 when Shannon reported that seven children became much less fretful, restless, and irritable when refined sugar was removed from their diet (Shannon, 1922). In the 1950's, Speer (1954; 1958) suggested that some food allergies could produce an "allergic tension-fatigue syndrome," a disorder of the nervous system. In support of Speer's hypothesis, Crook and colleagues (Crook, Harrison, Crawford, & Emerson, 1961; Crook, 1975a; Crook, 1975b) reported clinical cases of children with the symptoms of allergic tension-fatigue syndrome that were relieved when the offending foods were eliminated from their diets. However, it was Feingold (1968; 1975a; 1975b) who popularized the notion that certain food additives and colorings increased hyperactive behavior in sensitive children and allowed the notion that foods could affect behavior to gain scientific respectability.

Food Additives and Behavioral Disorders in Children

According to Feingold (1975a; 1975b), food additives, in particular synthetic and natural food colorings and flavorings, produced hyperkinesis (later termed 'hyperactivity') and learning disorders when ingested by susceptible children. Feingold (1968) derived this assumption from his treatment of adults who were sensitive to aspirin and aspirin-related products (salicylates) which occur naturally in some foods. These aspirin-sensitive clients reacted with allergic symptoms, such as allergic rhinitis, asthma, nasal polyps, pruritus (severe itching), urticaria (rash), edema, and headaches after the ingestion of salicylates. A salicylate-free diet was prescribed for adults with aspirin sensitivity (Feingold, 1968), with many clients reporting improvement in their allergic symptoms. However, because all clients did not respond favorably to the salicylate-free diet, Feingold (1968; 1975a; 1975b) claimed that thousands of artificial flavors and colorings might also result in allergic reactions.

Feingold (1968) argued that clients who did not respond to the salicylate-free diet were actually reacting to haptens (incomplete antigens) found in food flavorings and colorings, for which no skin tests exist. Although all food colorings and flavorings were suspect (Feingold, 1968; 1975a; 1975b), cyclamates found in artificial sweeteners and Yellow #5 (tartrazine) found in many drugs and foods were thought to be particularly likely to lead to allergic reactions. An additive-free diet became the treatment of choice for clients with one of four types of clinical symptoms: (1) clients with known aspirin sensitivity, (2) clients with nasal polyposis, (frequently associated with the ingestion of aspirin), (3) clients with allergy symptoms who do not react to allergy skin tests, and (4) clients who do react to allergy skin tests. This food-additive-free diet became known as the Kaiser-Permanente (K-P) diet, and the results from this dietary treatment led to Feingold's hypothesis that food colorings and flavorings, both natural and synthetic, occasionally produced behavioral disorders, including hyperactivity and learning disabilities in children (1975a; 1975b).

Feingold (1975a; 1975b) reported case studies where clients had displayed allergic-type symptoms and after following the K-P diet for several weeks reported a reduction in behavioral problems, such as hyperactivity, fidgeting, excitability, impulsiveness, and lack of concentration. Although no proposed mechanism was offered to explain this relationship between food additives and behavior, Feingold contended that food additives could be the primary cause of behavioral problems as a result of food intolerance, or the additives could be irritants to previous neurological damage. Hawley and Buckley (1974) asserted that clinical case studies had demonstrated that food dye allergy provoked hyperactivity in children and published instructions on how to test for food dye sensitivity sublingually. These researchers recommended the K-P diet as treatment for food sensitivities.

The anecdotal reports of a relationship between diet and behavior in children suggested an "on-again, off-again" pattern of hyperactivity according to whether certain prohibited foods had been ingested or not (Feingold, 1975b). According to Feingold (1975a; 1975b), 50% of hyperactive children placed on this additive-free diet showed marked improvement, with less hyperactivity and improved cognitive abilities. The other 50% of hyperactive children placed on this diet did not respond purportedly because of fetal exposure to food additives or other environmental toxicants, or failure to follow the diet strictly (Feingold, 1975a; 1975b). Feingold's hypotheses regarding diet and behavioral disorders gained wide acceptance in both the public and among medical practitioners.

Despite the seemingly positive effect Feingold's diet had on behavioral disorders in children, there were several problems with his early claims. First, the allegation that the 50% of children who failed to respond to his diet resulted from either fetal exposure or lack of compliance appeared to be a form of "circular reasoning" or begging the question. That is, Feingold appeared to discount disconfirming evidence regarding his theoretical model. Second, the claims that the 50% of children who apparently did respond to the Feingold diet did so because of factors consistent with his theoretical claims ignored the potential placebo effects his diet might engender, as well as possible expectancy biases of the parents and teachers who rated the children's behavior before, during, and after treatment with the K-P diet.

Given the potential problems with the early anecdotal reports regarding diet and behavior in children, researchers set out to test Feingold's hypotheses with controlled studies. Several early studies appeared to supported Feingold's assertions that food sensitivities played a role in hyperactive behavior in children (e.g., Conners, Goyette,

Southwick, Lees, & Andrulonis, 1976; Rapp, 1978; 1979). For example, Conners and his colleagues (Conners et al., 1976) conducted a controlled double-blind study where parents and teachers of 15 hyperkinetic children rated the children on several scales designed to measure behavioral problems considered characteristic of hyperkinesis. Behavioral ratings were obtained at baseline, the end of the first diet trial, and the end of the second diet trial. After the baseline ratings were completed, the children were placed on either the K-P diet or a control diet similar to the K-P diet in preparation time, food groupings, and overall appearance. The children were placed on each diet for four weeks, followed by the other diet for four weeks, so that each child received both diets. Parents were told that both diets might produce improvement in behavioral problems.

As part of the Conner et al. (1976) study, parents completed dietary questionnaires, performed 24-hour recalls on the children's consumption, and measured the frequency of consumption for certain foods. According to judgements made by Conner (Conner et al., 1976), five children significantly improved while on the K-P diet. Further results demonstrated that the teachers noted less hyperactive behavior when the children were on the K-P diet, but parents did not notice any differences in behavior between the K-P and control diets. Instead, the parents rated their children as less hyperactive when on either diet compared to the baseline ratings. According to the researchers, parents and teachers noted approximately 15% reduction in hyperactive symptoms while on the K-P diet compared to a 3% reduction in symptoms in the control diet. Conner et al. (p. 161) concluded that their results "strongly suggest that a diet free of most natural salicylates, artificial flavors, and artificial colors reduces the *perceived* hyperactivity of some children suffering from hyperkinetic impulse disorder" (italics added). Perceptions, however, are not always reliable, and because parents rated their children's behavior as no different on the K-P or control diet, yet improved on either diet compared to baseline, an expectancy effect produced when the researchers told the parents that either diet might improve the behavioral problems of the children can not be ruled out. Furthermore, although 15 children completed the study, 22 were lost to attrition, which may indicate that parents and teachers did not perceive any differences in behavior while on either diet for these children.

Rapp (1979) investigated the supposed relationship between food-additives and hyperactivity in a group of eleven children, all but one of whom had a positive allergy history. The children were on individualized diets for three to six months, and then were tested for allergy to 10-30 commonly ingested foods over the next one to three months using a provocative intradermal titration method. The provocative method involved injecting diluted food extracts interdermally, with the resulting wheal measured. The extracts were then increasingly diluted and injected interdermally until the wheal disappeared. According to the researchers, this modified form of skin testing was more accurate than the usual form of skin testing. Once the treatment dosage was established for each child, the children were treated with either sublingual dosages three times a day or subcutaneous treatment once daily. While undergoing treatment, the children were able to ingest foods previously found to cause hyperactive symptoms without any adverse symptoms.

Each child in the Rapp (1979) study was also given, under blind conditions, three bottles of extract identical in taste and appearance, two of which were slightly diluted and one of which was the treatment dilution for that particular child. Parents were asked to give the prescribed doses of extract according to a specific schedule, with each extract given for five to seven days. Five children out of eight were able to accurately select the placebo extracts not sufficiently diluted for a treatment extract. The three who chose the placebo extracts were considered to be non-allergic and were put on regular diets. Three children did not complete the study: Two developed behavioral problems during the extract testing and the parents withdrew the children from the study, and one child continued to ingest artificial food coloring throughout the investigation.

The provocative intradermal titration method has since come under fire as a reliable method of allergy testing (Ferguson, 1990; Jewett, Phil, Fein, & Greenberg, 1990). Jewett and colleagues (1990) found that when the intradermal titration method was used in a double-blind study, the treatments lacked validity, and positive results appeared to be the result of suggestion and chance. Since according to Rapp (1979), three children (out of eleven) found to be food sensitive through the provocative titration method were later regarded as non-food sensitive and placed back on regular diets, this unreliability appears to have been present in this study as well, possibly indicating that the children considered food-sensitive and treated with diluted extracts may not have been food sensitive after all. In addition, the child who did not complete the study due to continuous consumption of food colorings demonstrates just how difficult these individualized elimination diets can be without constant reading of food labels and attempts to find substitutes for many common ingredients.

The above suggests that although some early studies appeared to support the link between diet and hyperactivity, the actual findings were not compelling. Furthermore, many well-designed studies failed to support any link between food sensitivities and childhood behavior. For example, Harley and colleagues, in a double-blind trial that included objectively assessed hyperactivity measures in a lab setting as well as subjective ratings by parents and teachers did not find a relationship between food additives and hyperactive behavior (Harley et al., 1978). After a standardized interview and two weeks of baseline behavioral measurements, three samples for a total of 36 school-aged boys, previously diagnosed as hyperactive, were randomly assigned by a dietitian to either K-P or control diets, with all other persons involved in the project blind to conditions. The children were placed on each diet for three to four weeks, with neuropsychological, physical, and behavioral evaluations completed in the lab at the end of baseline and each diet trial. In addition, the parents and teachers of the children conducted weekly behavioral ratings. Harley and his associates also took steps to maximize compliance by meeting with the parents, sending dietitians into the homes, and removing all pre-existing food from the homes and delivering the groceries required for each week. Findings indicated that the efficacy of the Feingold K-P diet was not supported, with the highest frequency of positive effects from the diet reported by the parents. The frequency of positive effects of the diet dropped dramatically in teacher ratings and was nonexistent in the objective laboratory data. The results of this study implicate a possible expectancy effect from the parents rather than actual behavioral changes.

The public excitement over the proposed food-hyperactivity connection led to a search for other food substances that possibly affected the activity of children. Refined sugar became the next food villain to be investigated after books such as *Sugar Blues* (Dufty, 1975) and *Can Your Child Read? Is He Hyperactive?* (Crook, 1975a) were published (Benton, 1989; Christensen, 1996; Wolraich, 1988; Wolraich, Wilson, & White, 1995).

Sugar and Behavioral Disorders in Children

Refined sugar became a focus of studies investigating possible food influences on hyperactivity due to clinical case and anecdotal reports of decreased hyperactivity in children when refined sugar was removed during elimination diets (e.g., Crook, 1974; 1975b; Dufty, 1975; Rapp, 1978). Dufty (p. 136), based on anecdotal data, declared that "[a]ny diet which includes refined sugar and white flour, no matter what "scientific" name is applied to them [the sugar and flour], is dangerous." Furthermore, Cott (1977) suggested that along with lead poisoning, prenatal malnutrition, and birth complications, refined sugar is a cause of learning disabilities. According to Cott (1977, p. 91), "[s]ince many disturbed and learning disabled children are found to have either hypoglycemia, hyperinsulinism, or dysinsulinism, cane sugar and rapidly absorbed carbohydrates should be eliminated from their diets."

The proposed mechanism by which sugar affected hyperactivity and learning disabilities was through its effect on blood-glucose levels. All carbohydrates are converted to glucose after ingestion, which enters the blood stream and stimulates the release of insulin to transport the glucose to cells for energy and store the remainder of the glucose (Fishbein & Pease, 1994). Refined carbohydrates are broken down more quickly and lead to large amounts of glucose rapidly entering the blood stream. This large quantity of glucose causes a quick release of insulin in order to reduce the blood sugar level. Repeated ingestion of refined carbohydrates may lead to the release of an excessive amount of insulin in order to control the high glucose levels in the blood, which in turn produces a sharp drop in the blood glucose level (Fishbein & Pease). The brain reacts to low levels of glucose by releasing hormones, primarily adrenaline, prolactin, cortisol, and ACTH, which are also responsible for the "fight or flight response," often linked with irritable, agitated, and anxious states (see Fishbein & Pease, 1994, for an excellent review). Some researchers found that behavioral symptoms such as fatigue, irritability, nervousness, inability to concentrate, anxiety, and destructive outbursts were associated with rapid declines in blood sugar (e.g., Cooper & Pfeiffer, 1977; Fishbein, 1982; Johnson, Dorr, Swenson, & Service, 1980).

Cott (1977) hypothesized that this adult condition, referred to as 'functional reactive hypoglycemia' (FRH), also occurred in children, with the resulting low blood glucose levels contributing to learning disabilities and hyperactivity. This idea gained popularity after a study demonstrated the expected blood glucose patterns in hyperactive children after a glucose tolerance test (Langseth & Dowd, 1978). Early studies investigating the FRH and hyperactivity relationship found that hyperactive children (Goldman, Lerman, Contois, & Udall, 1986; Prinz, Roberts, & Hantman, 1980) and aggressive adults (Fishbein, 1982) exhibited calmer behavior after ingesting special diets that eliminated refined sugar and other refined carbohydrates from their diet. The successful "Twinkie Defense" used by Dan White, where excessive sugar intake was blamed for White's murder of two local politicians and resulted in a manslaughter rather than a first-degree murder conviction, brought the notion of sugar producing uncontrollable problem behavior into the limelight (Kanarek, 1994).

One of the earliest investigations to find evidence for the proposed refined sugar-hyperactivity association was a correlational study by Prinz and colleagues (Prinz et al., 1980). One group of children was obtained through media advertisements and consisted of children whose parents were concerned about their child's behavior and who met the criteria for hyperactivity, as determined by a psychologist. The control participants were recruited from the same community, also through advertisements. The daily food records for the children were maintained for a week by their mothers, and the children's activity was monitored through one-way mirrors before and after the food diaries were kept. Findings demonstrated that the two groups had similar food intake in respect to amount of sugar intake and type of foods eaten; however, the hyperactive group ate less in overall volume. Nonetheless, the hyperactive group differed from the control group when correlations were computed between dietary scores and behavior scores, with the hyperactive group displaying more destruction and aggression when they had ingested a ratio of high sugar intake to nutritional foods. The results suggested that the amount of sugar consumed, the ratio of sugar products to nutritional foods, and the ratio of carbohydrates to protein significantly affected the level of hyperactivity in young children.

A later study (Goldman et al., 1986) using a double-blind crossover design examined eight preschool children who had no history of hyperactivity. Each child was observed individually for one initial and two experimental visits, each one week apart. Before each of the two experimental visits, the children fasted the night before. During the experimental trial the children were observed for 15 minutes, then drank a glass of orange juice sweetened with 2 grams of sucrose or aspartame, and were then observed for another 90 minutes. The children were also assessed on structured tasks before the drink and then again at 30, 60, and 90 minutes after ingesting the drink. The researchers found that after drinking the sucrose mixture, the children had decreased performance and increased hyperactivity and distractibility, with the most pronounced effects 45-60 minutes after ingestion.

Fishbein (1982) investigated whether hypoglycemia could influence aggressive behavior in a prison population of young adults aged 16-28 years. The participants completed two surveys; one assessed the symptoms of hypoglycemia while the other assessed individually preferred foods. According to their mean scores on these two surveys, the inmates were assigned to either a hypoglycemic or nonhypoglycemic group. Once the inmates had been assigned to one of these two groups, they had their maladaptive behaviors assessed by the Hoffer-Osmond Diagnostic (HOD) Test and then assigned randomly to control or experimental groups, yielding four groups: hypoglycemic experimental, hypoglycemic control, nonhypoglycemic experimental, and nonhypoglycemic control. The experimental groups underwent special diets, designed to treat hypoglycemia by restricting refined carbohydrates for one month, then the participants were again assessed for problem behaviors with the HOD Test. Fishbein found that the hypoglycemic experimental group was significantly different from the other groups, with more drastic behavioral improvement while on the experimental diet than the other three groups.

Although some studies appeared to support a link between sugar and behavioral problems, other investigations did not support a relationship. For example, Gross (1984) examined 50 children whose mothers were convinced that their child was negatively affected by sugar. He utilized a double-blind procedure and had the children ingest a lemonade drink with either 75 grams of sucrose or saccharin for equivalent taste added. Mothers gave the challenge drinks at home and then rated their children's behavior for several hours afterwards. Each child received three trials per condition, with no particular time schedule except convenience for the mothers deciding when the trial would occur. Even considering the confounds of prior food consumption and the likelihood of expectancy effects due to the mother's certainty that their child was sensitive to sugar, Gross found no differences between the ingestion of sucrose compared to saccharin.

Notwithstanding the popular reception of food additives and refined sugar as causal factors in hyperactivity of children, many physicians and researchers expressed doubts that diet alone was the principal cause of the disorder (Bennett & Sherman, 1983). Often, pediatricians treated hyperactivity with a combination of pharmacotherapy, behavioral therapy, and dietary restrictions, hoping that the combination of treatment will provide more improvement than one specific treatment alone. Kanarek (1994) noted that studies investigating the FRH hypothesis often based diagnoses of hypoglycemia on symptoms self-reported by the participants rather than on actual glucose blood levels, making such diagnoses unreliable. An example of this self-report method is found in the study conducted by Fishbein (1982), who based her four groups within the prison population on self-reported symptoms of hypoglycemia.

The early and well-publicized research investigating the food additive/sugar and behavioral relationships had other serious methodological flaws as well (Benton, 1989; Christensen, 1996; Fishbein & Pease, 1994; Kanarek, 1994; Pescara-Kovach & Alexander, 1994; Wender, 1986; Wolraich, 1988; Wolraich, Lindgren, Stumbo, Stegink, Appelbaum, & Kiritsy, 1994; Wolraich et al., 1995), which are discussed in the following section. These methodological problems spurred later research with improved research design to further explore the proposed relationships between various food components and behavior.

Methodological Flaws of Early Diet-Behavior Research in Children

The early research of the relationship between food components and hyperactivity was plagued by several, serious methodological flaws, including basing causal claims on correlational data, uncontrolled studies, lack of placebo groups, expectancy biases, and problems with participant sampling (Benton, 1989; Christensen, 1996; Fishbein & Pease, 1994; Kanarek, 1994; Pescara-Kovach & Alexander, 1994; Wender, 1986; Wolraich, 1988; Wolraich et al., 1994; Wolraich et al., 1995). Correlational studies, which investigate possible associations between variables, are not intended to "prove" causation, since variables are uncontrolled and extraneous variables may exist, confounding the results (Christensen, 1996). The correlational study by Prinz and associates (1980) demonstrated a relationship between sugar and hyperactivity, but it is possible that the hyperactive children required an increased energy intake, leading to increased sugar consumption, rather than sugar causing hyperactivity (Christensen, 1996; Wolraich, 1988; Wolraich et al., 1995).

Uncontrolled studies and lack of placebo groups also question the validity of the findings of the earlier food and behavior studies (e.g., Conners et al., 1976; O'Banion & Greenberg, 1982; Rapp, 1978; 1979). When experimental groups do not have an appropriate control group, many extraneous variables may make clear interpretation of the findings impossible. Extraneous events that may have occurred during the same time period as the study, placebo effects, and participant or researcher bias are just a few of the confounding variables that could affect the results (Benton, 1989; Christensen, 1996; Wolraich et al., 1995).

Many early studies failed to consider the difficulty of generalizing results from diet-behavior studies across extremely small samples and distinct populations. Samples of less than 20 participants were common (e.g., Goldman et al., 1986; Milich & Pelham, 1986; O'Banion & Greenberg, 1982; Rapp, 1979; Wolraich et al., 1985). In addition, studies have been conducted with very disparate populations, such as diagnosed hyperactive children (e.g., Connors et al., 1976; Harley et al., 1978; Prinz et al., 1980), children with normal activity levels (e.g., Goldman et al., 1986), aggressive adults who are in prison (Fishbein, 1982), and adults who are suspected of being food-allergic (e.g., O'Banion & Greenberg, 1982). Such distinct samples lead to difficulties interpreting any possible overall diet-behavioral link (Kanarek, 1994).

Expectancy effects, where either the expectancy of the participant or researcher can bias the outcome of a study, is another methodological issue not considered by early researchers (Benton, 1989; Christensen, 1996; Fishbein & Pease, 1994; Pescara-Kovach & Alexander, 1994). Open studies are well-known for researcher and participant bias since everyone knows that all participants are receiving the treatment hypothesized to be effective, or in the case of the refined sugar studies hypothesized to be the causal factor of problem behavior, so both the researchers and the participants expect some type of behavioral influence to result from the ingestion of the food component in question (Christensen, 1996). According to Christensen (1996), expectancy effects should be anticipated when conducting research that explores diet-behavioral relationships, and study design should control for this possible confounding effect.

Earlier study designs (e.g., Crook, 1974; Rapp, 1978) that relied on parent and teacher behavioral ratings of the children may be misleading because of the rater's preconceived notions about a sugar-behavior link (Benton, 1989; Christensen, 1996; Pescara-Kovach & Alexander, 1994). For instance, Rapp (1978) relied upon parent ratings of activity during the open-design special diet period of his study, a methodology which may have biased the study toward supporting a sugar-behavior relationship, especially when one considers that two children reacted to control substances during the sublingual testing.

Two methods recommended to control for expectancy effects include the double-blind placebo controlled experiment and the challenge experiment (Christensen, 1996; Fishbein & Pease, 1994; Kanarek, 1994; Wolraich, 1988). The double-blind placebo controlled experiment prevents the researcher or participant from knowing which treatment is received. This type of experiment controls for placebo effects, researcher biases, and expectancy effects. Challenge studies typically remove the suspected food from a participant's diet for several days or weeks, then re-introduce the suspected food at periods unknown to the participant. This form of experiment also controls for the expectancy effect (Christensen, 1996). When researchers investigate sugar intake, a substitute sweetener such as aspartame is often used to prevent the participant from discovering when sugar has been added to the diet. Other methodological issues unique to diet and behavior research include the necessity to separate nutritional from nonnutritional factors, to consider prior nutritional status, to consider the expected temporal conditions of the behavioral effect, to decide if whole food or a specific nutrient is to be studied, to decide the dose level, and to consider whether a wash-out period is required to control for the effect of previous food intake (Christensen, 1996; Kanarek, 1994).

Later research using improved study design, such as the double-blind placebo controlled experiment or the challenge tests, found that the association between sugar and hyperactivity was likely dubious. In fact, although most recent studies find no differences in activity between treatment and control groups of children receiving sugar or food additives (e.g., Ferguson, 1986; Gross et al., 1987; Milich & Pelham, 1986; Wolraich et al., 1994; Wolraich, Milich, Stumbo, & Schultz, 1985; Wolraich, Stumbo, Milich, Chenard, & Schultz, 1986), one study actually found *improved* performance and decreased activity with sugar intake (Benton, Brett, & Brain, 1987).

A review by Milich, Wolraich, and Lindgren (1986) of research to that date indicated that although the early correlational studies showed a relationship of sugar ingestion and behavior, most of the dietary challenge studies found no differences in behavior and a few studies found that sugar improved behavior and performance. More recently, a meta-analysis (Wolraich et al., 1995) of controlled, double-blind studies investigating the refined sugar-hyperactivity association found no evidence that refined sugar affected the behavior or cognitive performance of children. These researchers stated that the strong belief of parents in this link between sugar and problem behavior might be the result of expectancy effects.

Conclusion

Despite the contemporary research (e.g., Benton et al., 1987; Gross et al., 1987; Milich & Pelham, 1986; Wolraich et al., 1994; Wolraich et al., 1995) that suggests that food additives and/or refined sugar do not generally precipitate hyperactivity in children, popular belief in this food-behavior relationship persists. For example, fairly recent books (Lavin, 1989; Taylor, 1990) promote the Feingold Diet, as well as behavior modification, for the treatment of hyperactivity in children. Colquboun (1994) discussed the Feingold Diet as part of the rehabilitation of hyperactive children, with reports of several studies undertaken in the U. K. in 1979 and 1980 given as evidence of effectiveness. However, it should be noted that these studies were open, with parents rating their children's behavior or personnel rating the behavior of a very small institutionalized population. These open studies likely produced expectancy effects that could have been responsible for the perceived decrease in hyperactivity. Crook (1994), Brenner (1994), and Ferguson (1990) all have recently affirmed their belief in the relationship between food additives and/or sugar and behavior in people with food sensitivity.

According to many of the contemporary researchers in the field (Benton, 1989; Christensen, 1996; Wender, 1986; Wolraich et al., 1994, Wolraich et al., 1985; Wolraich et al., 1995), when children undergo food-additive or sucrose testing under double-blind procedures, the relationship between diet and behavior almost disappears. Benton (1989) and Kanarek (1994) suggest that a few children may be sensitive to food additives or sucrose that results in problem behavior due simply to the idiosyncrasies of humans. As Kanarek (1994, p. 533) stated, "At best, only a small percentage of hyperactive children may be adversely affected by food additives." Indeed, Ferguson (1990) cautioned that often doctors and patients are quick to blame food sensitivities for symptoms that often are psychiatric in nature. Parker and colleagues (1991) echoed this advice. Another warning that should be heeded by practitioners is the powerful placebo effect. A study that explored the effectiveness of methylphenidate, a medication used in treatment of Attention Deficit Disorder, demonstrated that 18% of the children tested responded as well to a placebo as other children responded to the active medication according to assessments of behavior (Ullmann & Sleator, 1986). The researchers proclaimed that had a placebo group not been included in the study design, these placebo-responders would have been considered responders to the medication. Ullmann and her associates strongly emphasize the importance of double-blind, controlled research designs to prevent this type of confound. This warning should also be heeded by the diet-behavior researchers when conducting future studies.

DIET, DEPRESSION, AND OBESITY

The literature on diet and childhood behavioral disorders exemplifies the common result of research on the psychoactive properties of foods–well controlled studies find little or no evidence that the food substance produces clinically significant effects on mood or behavior. However, there are examples where a food substance's purported psychoactive effects are supported in well-conducted research studies. One of the most widely accepted relationships between food and mood is that between the large neutral amino acid (LNAA) tryptophan and depression (Christensen, 1996). The biosynthesis of the brain neurotransmitter serotonin (5-HT) is dependent on dietary tryptophan, which cannot be produced endogenously (Cowen, Parry-Billings, & Newsholme, 1989; Spring et al., 1987; Wurtman & Wurtman, 1989; Young, 1993). Therefore, in order for 5-HT to be synthesized an individual must maintain a diet that contains a sufficient amount of tryptophan. This raises the possibility that diets that raise or lower the level of plasma tryptophan may also affect 5-HT levels. Because 5-HT plays an important role in mood regulation, a potential link between tryptophan and mood has been the focus of much research (Cowen et al., 1989; Fernstrom & Wurtman, 1971a, 1971b, 1972; Lieberman, Wurtman, & Chew, 1986; Young, 1993).

Prior to reviewing the literature on tryptophan and mood, it is important to understand the conditions that must exist for diet to affect the synthesis of a neurotransmitter. Christensen (1996) provides an excellent summary of the five specific conditions that determine whether diet will affect neurotransmitter production: (1) the plasma levels of a precursor must be able to fluctuate with dietary intake, (2) there cannot be an absolute blood-brain barrier so that the precursor can travel to the brain's extracellular space, (3) the mechanism responsible for the transport of the precursor to the brain cannot be fully saturated at normal plasma concentrations, (4) the enzyme responsible for transforming the precursor into the neurotransmitter cannot be saturated, and (5) the enzyme that catalyzes the synthesis of the neurotransmitter cannot be subject to feedback inhibition. If any of these five conditions are not met, then the precursor (i.e., food substance) will not affect neurotransmitter production. For example, an increase in the availability to the precursor for the catecholamines, tyrosine, does not consistently result in an increase in catecholamine production because of feedback inhibition under specific circumstances (cf., Sved, 1983). Production of 5-HT, however, appears to meet all of these conditions.

Biosynthesis of 5-HT

Figure 1 presents a diagram of the biosynthesis of 5-HT from tryptophan. First, tryptophan is converted to 5-hydroxytryptophan (5-HTP) by the enzyme tryptophan hydroxylase. Remember that one condition that must exist for diet to affect neurotransmitter synthesis is that the enzyme responsible for transforming the precursor (in this case tryptophan) into a neurotransmitter (here 5-HT) must not be saturated. Studies in both rats (Sved, 1983) and humans (Young, 1986) have demonstrated that tryptophan hydroxylase is only about half saturated under normal circumstances. This suggests that increases in brain tryptophan can increase the synthesis of 5-HT as much as twofold (Young, 1986). As Figure 1 also indicates, 5-HTP is converted to 5-HT by the enzyme 5-HTP decarboxylase. Because of the dependence of 5-HT biosynthesis on tryptophan, studies have clearly dem-

FIGURE 1. Serotonin Synthesis

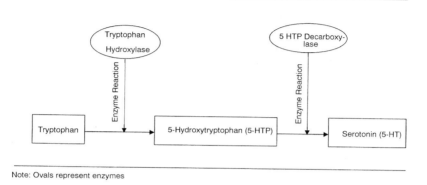

Note: Ovals represent enzymes

onstrated that brain 5-HT levels are responsive to brain tryptophan levels (e.g., Fernstrom & Wurtman, 1971a).

Diets That Produce Changes in Brain Tryptophan Levels

As an amino acid, the body's entire supply of tryptophan is dependent on dietary protein. One might reasonably conclude, therefore, that increases in protein consumption would also increase 5-HT production due to the corresponding increase in available tryptophan. In reality, studies have demonstrated that brain tryptophan and 5-HT actually *decrease* following a protein rich meal (Fernstrom & Wurtman, 1972). This seemingly paradoxical effect results from the fact that the transport system that carries LNAAs across the blood-brain barrier is competitive. Because protein contains very small amounts of tryptophan (i.e., 1%-1.5%) compared to the other LNAAs (i.e., leucine, isoleucine, valine, tyrosine, and phenylalanine; 25%), a high-protein meal results in a decrease in brain tryptophan relative to its competitors. In other words, in the presence of increased availability of LNAAs, tryptophan is crowded out by other LNAAs and as a result brain levels of tryptophan decline.

Because tryptophan competes with other LNAAs for transportation across the blood-brain barrier, the ratio of tryptophan to the total quantity of LNAAs, rather than the absolute plasma concentration of tryptophan, determines brain levels of tryptophan (Lieberman et al.,

1986). A protein-rich meal increases the denominator of the tryptophan/LNAA ratio and as a result the ratio becomes small and levels of brain tryptophan decline. How can one, therefore, significantly alter the tryptophan/LNAA ratio? One method involves administering a relatively large dose of tryptophan (i.e., > 500mg) to individuals either orally or by injection (see Christensen, 1996, for an excellent review of research methodologies in this area). Another approach involves examining participants who are given an amino acid cocktail that is either depleted of or supplemented with tryptophan. Studies using each of these methods of altering available tryptophan have typically found significant relationships between tryptophan availability, mood, and behavior (Christensen, 1996). However, these methods of altering the tryptophan/LNAA ratio are not likely representative of diets actually consumed by obese individuals.

One approach to altering the tryptophan/LNAA ratio that may have applications to obesity involves the consumption of a carbohydrate-rich and protein poor meal (Lieberman et al., 1986). Proponents of the addictions model of obesity often point to high carbohydrate foods as likely to produce a psychoactive response in obese individuals (e.g., Sheppard, 1993). Although neither tryptophan nor the other LNAAs are present in a pure carbohydrate meal, high carbohydrate meals alter the tryptophan/LNAA ratio as a result of the increased secretion of insulin such meals produce. Because insulin lowers the plasma levels of other LNAAs relative to tryptophan, high-carbohydrate meals increase the tryptophan/LNAA ratio and levels of brain tryptophan (Fernstrom & Wurtman, 1972).

One might be tempted to conclude that because consuming a carbohydrate rich, protein poor diet leads to increased 5-HT production that chronic consumption of such a diet would affect mood and behavior. However, research has challenged the notion that a high carbohydrate diet significantly alters mood or behavior. Christensen (1996), for instance, provides a review of studies that examines the effects of a carbohydrate-rich diet on mood and concludes that "these results clearly indicate that the mood-altering effects of carbohydrates are either very weak or nonexistent" (p. 81). If a high carbohydrate, protein poor meal is associated with increased brain tryptophan levels in laboratory studies, then why have researchers not found a relationship between high carbohydrate consumption and increased 5-HT biosynthesis in humans?

Several factors are likely responsible for the insignificant relationship between a high-carbohydrate diet and mood. First, between a 50% and 100% increase in the tryptophan/LNAA ratio is required to produce a significant change in 5-HT biosynthesis–a change that cannot occur in a normal diet (Curzon & Sarna, 1984). In fact, in laboratory studies where meals are created to contain only carbohydrate, the tryptophan/LNAA ratio is not altered sufficiently to result in significant changes in 5-HT biosynthesis (Christensen, 1996). Second, a meal which contains even a small amount of protein (i.e., approximately 5%) will prevent the rise of brain tryptophan levels (Fernstrom, 1988). Few foods in the American diet contain less than 5% protein. Even if pure sucrose were consumed, recent data suggests that feedback mechanisms connected to the serotonergic neurons limit the effect dietary variables can exert on neurotransmission (Christensen, 1996). As a result of these limiting factors, any change in 5-HT biosynthesis occurring as the result of carbohydrate consumption is likely to be either nonexistent or small and will occur only under specific circumstances. Therefore, in the context of the effects of carbohydrate consumption on 5-HT biosynthesis, the premise of the addictions model of obesity that the body responds to food identical to the way it reacts to psychoactive drugs such as antidepressants (e.g., Yeary, 1987) appears to be unsupported by the literature.

Carbohydrate Craving and Obesity

Although a high carbohydrate meal does not appear to be related to mood or behavior in most studies, it has been argued that among obese individuals there exists a clinically important subgroup who have strong cravings for high carbohydrate foods (e.g., Caballero, 1987; Lieberman et al., 1986; Wurtman & Suffes, 1996). Fernstrom (1988) outlines the theoretical model underlying the proposed relationship between carbohydrate consumption and mood regulation among carbohydrate cravers. First, the consumption of carbohydrate-rich foods is said to alter the tryptophan/LNAA ratio so as to increase brain tryptophan levels and stimulate 5-HT biosynthesis. Second, when feedback mechanisms detect the increased release of 5-HT they inhibit the subsequent ingestion of carbohydrates and favor the intake of protein. Because increased protein consumption lowers brain tryptophan and 5-HT biosynthesis, feedback mechanisms cause the individual to again crave carbohydrates. In essence, therefore, carbohydrate cravers are using carbohydrate intake to regulate 5-HT biosynthesis and ultimately their mood. This model also suggests that the periodic, excessive intake of carbohydrate rich foods results in excessive total caloric intake and contributes to the development and maintenance of obesity.

Several studies have documented that many obese individuals report craving carbohydrate rich food and consume most of their snacks in the form of carbohydrates (e.g., Caballero, 1987; Lieberman et al., 1986; Wurtman et al., 1981). Also, support for the idea that consumption of high carbohydrate foods serves as a method to regulate mood via 5-HT biosynthesis comes from some studies which demonstrate that drugs which increase serotonergic neurotransmission (e.g., d-fenfluramine) produce decreases in carbohydrate intake, particularly during snacking (e.g., Wurtman et al., 1985). Because of these early studies and the belief of many obese individuals that they cannot control their carbohydrate consumption, the notion that carbohydrate craving serves an important role in the etiology and maintenance of obesity has gained wide appeal (e.g., Wurtman, 1983; Wurtman, 1986; Wurtman & Suffes, 1996).

There are numerous problems, however, with the basic premises of the carbohydrate craving model (Fernstrom, 1988). First, it is quite difficult to define who is a carbohydrate craver. Previous studies of carbohydrate cravers generally screen participants on the basis of their self-identified preference for high carbohydrate, protein poor foods. However, almost all such foods are also high in fat, are sweet, and are often visually appealing, which makes it difficult to identify which characteristic is the primary stimulus for the participant's selection (Fernstrom, 1988). Similarly, Drewnowski and colleagues (Drewnowski, Kurth, Holden-Wiltse, & Saari, 1992) have demonstrated that obese women prefer both high carbohydrate and high fat foods, while obese men tend to crave high protein and high fat foods. The carbohydrate craving model has difficulty explaining the gender difference in preferences and why obese females actually crave foods that are fat, sweet, or both.

Another problem with the carbohydrate craving model of obesity is that, as was reviewed above, high carbohydrate meals are unlikely to significantly alter 5-HT biosynthesis. Nearly all high carbohydrate foods used in studies of carbohydrate cravings contain levels of protein that will block any diet induced change in 5-HT synthesis (Fernstrom, 1988). As a result, the participants could not have been prompted to eat high carbohydrate foods because of their ability to increase 5-HT production. Also, the results of several studies that examined the effects of either serotinergic drugs or tryptophan on carbohydrate cravings are counter to the carbohydrate craving model (e.g., Hrboticky, Leiter, & Anderson, 1985; Toornvliet, Pijl, Hopman, Elte-de Wever, & Meinders, 1996).

A particularly damaging problem with the carbohydrate craving model comes from studies that fail to demonstrate that carbohydrate craving participants actually improve their mood following a carbohydrate-rich meal. For instance, Toornvliet and colleagues (Toornvliet et al., 1997) examined the psychological and metabolic responses of carbohydrate craving and noncarbohydrate craving obese individuals to carbohydrate, fat, or protein-rich meals in a double-blind, randomized research design. Both carbohydrate craving and noncarbohydrate craving participants had similar psychological and metabolic responses to each meal type. Also, carbohydrate craving participants did not significantly improve their mood through consumption of a high carbohydrate snack. These researchers conclude that, at least from a therapeutic point of view, carbohydrate craving was not a valuable concept to maintain in obesity research.

Several additional problems with the carbohydrate craving model of obesity exist (cf., Fernstrom, 1988); however, these should suffice to demonstrate that carbohydrates do not act as potent, psychoactive drugs as has been claimed by the addictions model of obesity. Although certain food substances (e.g., tryptophan) may cause modest changes in mood in specific circumstances (e.g., in the context of a protein poor meal), this does not provide a fruitful explanation for the complex problem of obesity.

CONCLUSIONS

This paper addressed the question of whether foods act as potent psychoactive drugs as has been claimed by adherents of the addictions model of obesity (e.g., Yeary, 1987). We conclude that although, under certain circumstances, some food substances may have subtle effects on mood and behavior, the effects of food are quite different from that of psychoactive drugs such as nicotine and alcohol. Moreover, the diets consumed by obese individuals do not typically conform to the prerequisites for diets that alter neurotransmitter biosynthesis. Although the theoretical model underlying the addictions model of obesity appears to be critically flawed, that does not necessarily mean that therapies based on this model are ineffective. However, there is at least some evidence that treatments based on the addictions model are no more effective than other treatments and may have unexpected, negative side effects (Parham, 1995).

Convincing patients that certain foods are highly addictive and that they are powerless to control their compulsive eating may promote feelings of deprivation and low self-efficacy. Furthermore, patients may ignore important components of their disordered eating if they believe that the addictions model provides a sufficient explanation of their obesity. Also, the addictions model notion that there is no cure for the compulsive eating may be a false claim (Fairburn & Wilson, 1993; Parham, 1995) and may lead to unnecessary pessimism regarding the likelihood of returning to a normal, healthy lifestyle. Finally, because the addictions model of obesity appears to be based on several highly questionable premises, adherence to this model may inhibit therapists from understanding actual controlling variables in their patient's condition (Parham, 1995). Taken together, these potential side effects of the addictions model of obesity treatment suggest the possibility that this model may actually exacerbate the patient's condition.

REFERENCES

American Psychiatric Association (1987). *Diagnostic and statistical manual of mental disorders* (3rd edition, revised). Washington, DC: Author.

Bennett, F. C., & Sherman, R. (1983). Management of childhood "hyperactivity" by primary care physicians. *Developmental and Behavioral Pediatrics, 4*, 88-93.

Benton, D. (1989). Sugar and children's behavior. In L. Pulkkinen & J. M. Ramirez (Eds.), *Aggression in children* (pp. 3-29). Sevilla, Spain: Publicaciones de la Universidad de Sevilla.

Benton, D., Brett, V., & Brain, P. F. (1987). Glucose improves attention and reaction to frustration in children. *Biological Psychology, 24*, 95-100.

Brenner, A. (1994). Sugar and children's behavior [Letter to the editor]. *The New England Journal of Medicine, 330*, p. 1902.

Caballero, B. (1987). Brain serotonin and carbohydrate cravings in obesity. *International Journal of Obesity, 11* (Suppl. 3), 179-183.

Christensen, L. (1996). *Diet-behavior relationships: Focus on depression*. Washington, DC: American Psychological Association.

Colquboun, I. (1994). Attention deficit/hyperactivity disorder–A dietary/nutritional approach. *Therapeutic Care and Education, 3*, 159-172.

Cooper, A., & Pfeiffer, C. (1977). *Functional hypoglycemia: Ubiquitous malady, Vol. III.* Princeton, NJ: Brain Bioresearch Center.

Conners, C. K., Goyette, C. H., Southwick, D. A., Lees, J. M., & Andrulonis, P. A. (1976). Food additives and hyperkinesis: A controlled double-blind experiment. *Pediatrics, 58,* 154-166.

Cott, A. (1977). Treatment of learning disabilities. In R. J. William & D. K. Kalita (Eds.). *A physician's handbook on orthomolecular medicine* (pp. 90-91). New York: Pergamon Press.

Cowen, P. J., Parry-Billings, M., & Newsholme, E. A. (1989). Decreased plasma tryptophan levels in major depression. *Journal of Affective Disorders, 16,* 27-31.

Crook, W. G. (1974). An alternative method of managing the hyperactive child. *Pediatrics, 54,* 656.

Crook, W. G. (1975a). *Can your child read? Is he hyperactive?* Jackson, TN: Pedicenter Press.

Crook, W. G. (1975b). Food allergy–The great masquerader. *Pediatric Clinics of North America, 22,* 227-238.

Crook, W. G. (1994). Sugar and children's behavior [Letter to the editor]. *The New England Journal of Medicine, 330,* 1902.

Crook, W. G., Harrison, W. W., Crawford, S. E., & Emerson, B. S. (1961). Systemic manifestations due to allergy: Report of fifty patients and a review of the literature on the subject. *Pediatrics, 27,* 790-799.

Curzon, G., & Sarna, G. S. (1984). Tryptophan transport into the brain: Newer findings and older ones reconsidered. In H. G. Schlossberger, W. Kochen, B. Linzen, & H. Steinhart (Eds.), *Progress in tryptophan and serotonin research* (pp. 145-160). New York: Walter de Gruyter.

Drewnowski, A., Kurth, C., Holden-Wiltse, J., & Saari, J. (1992). Food preferences in human obesity: Carbohydrates versus fats. *Appetite, 18,* 207-221.

Dufty, W. (1975). *Sugar blues.* Radnor, PA: Chilton.

Fairburn, C. G., & Wilson, G. T. (1993). *Binge eating: Nature, assessment, and treatment.* New York: The Guilford Press.

Feingold, B. F. (1968). Recognition of food additives as a cause of symptoms of allergy. *Annals of Allergy, 26,* 309-313.

Feingold, B. F. (1975a). Hyperkinesis and learning disabilities linked to artificial food flavors and colors. *American Journal of Nursing, 75,* 797-803.

Feingold, B. F. (1975b). *Why your child is hyperactive.* New York: Random House.

Ferguson, H. B. (1986). Double-blind challenge studies of behavioral and cognitive effects of sucrose-aspartame ingestion in normal children. *Nutrition Reviews, 44(Suppl.),* 144-150.

Ferguson, H. B. (1990). Food sensitivity or self-deception? *The New England Journal of Medicine, 323,* 476-478.

Fernstrom, J. D. (1988). Tryptophan, serotonin, and carbohydrate appetite: Will the real carbohydrate craver please stand up! *Journal of Nutrition, 118,* 1417-1419.

Fernstrom, J. D., & Wurtman, R. J. (1971a). Brain serotonin content: Increase following ingestion of carbohydrate diet. *Science, 171,* 1023-1025.

Fernstrom, J. D., & Wurtman, R. J. (1971b). Brain serotonin content: Physiological dependence on plasma tryptophan levels. *Science, 171,* 1023-1025.

Fernstrom, J. D., & Wurtman, R. J. (1972). Brain serotonin content: Physiological regulation by plasma neutral amino acids. *Science, 178*, 414-416.

Fishbein, D. H. (1982). The contribution of refined carbohydrate consumption to maladaptive behaviors. *Orthomolecular Psychiatry, 11*, 17-25.

Fishbein, D. H., & Pease, S. E. (1994). Diet, nutrition, and aggression. In M. Hillbrand & N. J. Pallone (Eds.), *The psychobiology of aggression: Engines, measurement, and control* (pp. 117-144). New York: Hawthorn Press.

Goldman, J. A., Lerman, R. H., Contois, J. H., & Udall, J. N. (1986). Behavioral effects of sucrose on preschool children. *Journal of Abnormal Child Psychology, 14*, 565-577.

Gross, M. D. (1984). Effect of sucrose on hyperkinetic children. *Pediatrics, 74*, 876-878.

Gross, M. D., Tofanelli, R. A., Butzirus, S. M., & Snodgrass, E. W. (1987). The effect of diets rich in and free from additives on the behavior of children with hyperkinetic and learning disorders. *American Academy of Child and Adolescent Psychiatry, 26*, 53-55.

Harley, J. P., Ray, R. S., Tomasi, L., Eichman, P. L., Matthews, C. G., Chun, R., Cleeland, C. S., & Traisman, E. (1978). Hyperkinesis and food additives: Testing the Feingold hypothesis. *Pediatrics, 61*, 818-828.

Hawley, C., & Buckley, R. (1974). Food dyes and hyperkenetic (sic) children. *Academic Theory, 10*, 27-32.

Hrboticky, N., Leiter, L. A., & Anderson, G. H. (1985). Effects of L-tryptophan on short term food intake in lean men. *Nutrition Research, 5*, 595-607.

Jewett, D. L., Phil, D., Fein, G., & Greenberg, M. H. (1990). A double-blind study of symptom provocation to determine food sensitivity. *The New England Journal of Medicine, 32*, 429-433.

Johnson, D. D., Dorr, K. E., Swensen, W. M., & Service, J. (1980). Reactive hypoglycemia. *Journal of the American Medical Association, 243*, 1151-1155.

Kanarek, R. B. (1994). Nutrition and violent behavior. In A. J. Reiss, Jr., K. A. Miczek, & J. A. Roth (Eds.), *Understanding and preventing violence: Vol. 2. Biobehavioral influences* (pp. 515-538). Washington, DC: National Academy Press.

Kayloe, J. C. (1993). Food addiction. *Psychotherapy, 30*, 269-275.

Langseth, L., & Dowd, J. (1978). Glucose tolerance and hyperkinesis. *Food and Cosmetics Toxicology, 16*, 120-133.

Lavin, P. (1989). *Parenting the overactive child*. Lanham, MD: Madison Books.

Lieberman, H. R., Spring, B. J., & Garfield, G. S. (1986). The behavioral effects of food constituents: Strategies used in studies of amino acids, protein, carbohydrates, and caffeine. *Nutrition Reviews, 44*(Suppl.), 61-70.

Lieberman, H. R., Wurtman, J. J., & Chew, B. (1986). Changes in mood after carbohydrate consumption among obese individuals. *American Journal of Clinical Nutrition, 44*, 772-778.

Milich, R., & Pelham, W. E. (1986). Effects of sugar ingestion on the classroom and playgroup behavior of Attention Deficit Disordered boys. *Journal of Consulting and Clinical Psychology, 54*, 714-718.

Milich, R., Wolraich, M., & Lindgren, S. (1986). Sugar and hyperactivity: A critical review of empirical findings. *Clinical Psychology Review, 6,* 493-513.

Minirth, F. (1991). *Love hunger: Recovery from food addiction.* NY: Fawcett Books.

O'Banion, D. R., & Greenberg, M. R. (1982). Behavioral effects of food sensitivity. *International Journal of Biosocial Research, 3,* 55-68.

Overeaters Anonymous. (1997-1998). Group survey reveals needs and expectations of members. *A Step Ahead* [On-line], *7.* Available: http://www.overeatersanony mous.org /stephead.htm.

Neims, A. H. (1986). Individuality in the response to dietary constituents: Some lessons from drugs. *Nutrition Reviews, 44,* (Suppl., May), 237-241.

Parham, E. S. (1995). Compulsive eating: Applying a medical addiction model. In T. B. VanItallie and A. P. Simopoulos (Eds.), *Obesity: New directions in assessment and management.* Philadelphia, PA: The Charles Press, Publishers.

Parker, S. L., Garner, D. M., Leznoff, A., Sussman, G. L., Tarlo, S. M., & Krondl, M. (1991). Psychological characteristics of patients with reported adverse reactions to foods. *International Journal of Eating Disorders, 10,* 433-439.

Pescara-Kovach, L. A., & Alexander, K. (1994). The link between food ingested and problem behavior: Fact or fallacy? *Behavioral Disorders, 19,* 142-148.

Prinz, R. J., Roberts, W. A., & Hantman, E. (1980). Dietary correlates of hyperactive behavior in children. *Journal of Consulting and Clinical Psychology, 48,* 760-769.

Rapp, D. (1978). Does diet affect hyperactivity? *Journal of Learning Disabilities, 11,* 383-389.

Rapp, D. (1979). Food allergy treatment for hyperkinesis. *Journal of Learning Disabilities, 12,* 42-50.

Rounsaville, B. J., Spitzer, R. L., & Williams, J. B. W. (1986). Proposed changes in DSM-III substance use disorders: Description and rationale. *American Journal of Psychiatry, 143,* 463-468.

Shannon, W. R. (1922). Neuropathologic manifestations in infants and children as a result of anaphylactic reaction to foods contained in their dietary. *American Journal of Diseases in Children, 24,* 89-94.

Sheppard, K. (1989). *Food addiction: The body knows.* Deerfield Beach, FL: Health Communications, Inc.

Sheppard, K. (1993). *Food addiction: The body knows* (revised and expanded edition). Deerfield Beach, FL: Health Communications, Inc.

Speer, F. (1954). The allergic tension-fatigue syndrome. *Pediatric Clinics of North America, 1,* 1029-1037.

Speer, F. (1958). The allergic tension-fatigue syndrome in children. *International Archives of Allergy and Applied Immunology, 12,* 207.

Spring, B., Chiodo, J., & Bowen, D. J. (1987). Carbohydrates, tryptophan, and behavior: A methodological review. *Psychological Bulletin, 102,* 234-256.

Sved, A. F. (1983). Precursor control of the function of monoaminergic neurons. In R. J. Wurtman & J. J. Wurtman (Eds.), *Nutrition and the brain* (vol. 6, pp. 223-275). New York: Raven Press.

Taylor, J. F. (1990). *Helping your hyperactive child.* Rocklin, CA: Prima Publishing & Communications.

Toornvliet, A. C., Pijl, H., Hopman, E., Elte-de Wever, B. M., & Meinders, A. E.

(1996). Serotoninergic drug-induced weight loss in carbohydrate craving obese patients. *International Journal of Obesity and Related Metabolic Disorders, 20,* 917-920.

Toornvliet, A. C., Pijl, H., Tuinenburg, J. C., Elte-de Wever, B. M., Pieters, M. S., Frolich, M., Onkenhout, W., & Meinders, A. E. (1997). Psychological and metabolic responses of carbohydrate craving obese patients to carbohydrate, fat, and protein-rich meals. *International Journal of Obesity and Related Metabolic Disorders, 21,* 860-864.

Ullmann, R. K., & Sleator, E. K. (1986). Responders, nonresponders, and placebo responders among children with Attention Deficit Disorder: Importance of a blinded placebo evaluation. *Clinical Pediatrics, 25,* 594-599.

Vandereycken, W. (1990). The addiction model in eating disorders: Some critical remarks and a selected bibliography. *International Journal of Eating Disorders, 9,* 95-101.

Wender, E. H. (1986). The food additive-free diet in the treatment of behavior disorders: A review. *Journal of Development and Behavioral Pediatrics, 7,* 35-42.

Wilson, G. T. (1991). The addiction model of eating disorders: A critical analysis. *Advances in Behavior Research and Therapy, 13,* 27-72.

Wilson, G. T. (1999). Eating disorders and addiction. *Drugs & Society, 15,* 87-101.

Wolraich, M. L. (1988). Sugar intolerance: Is there evidence for its effects on behavior in children. *Annals of Allergy, 61(part 2),* 58-62.

Wolraich, M. L., Lindgren, S. D., Stumbo, P. J., Steglink, L. D., Appelbaum, M. I., & Kiritsy, M. C. (1994). Effects of diets high in sucrose or aspartame on the behavior and cognition performance of children. *The New England Journal of Medicine, 330,* 301-307.

Wolraich, M., Milich, R., Stumbo, P., & Schultz, F. (1985). Effects of sucrose ingestion on the behavior of hyperactive boys. *The Journal of Pediatrics, 106,* 675-682.

Wolraich, M. L., Stumbo, P., Milich, R., Chenard, C., & Schultz, F. (1986). Dietary characteristics of hyperactive and control boys. *Journal of the American Dietetic Association, 86,* 500-504.

Wolraich, M. L., Wilson, D. B., & White, J. W. (1995). The effect of sugar on behavior or cognition in children: A meta-analysis. *JAMA, 274,* 1617-1621.

Wurtman, J. J. (1983). *The carbohydrate craver's diet.* Boston, MA: Houghton Mifflin.

Wurtman, J. J. (1986). *Managing your mind and mood through food.* New York: Rawson Associates.

Wurtman, J. J. & Suffes, S. (1996). *Serotonin solution.* New York: Fawcett Columbine.

Wurtman, J. J., Wurtman, R. J., Growdon, J. H., Henry, P., Lipscomb, A., & Zeisel, S. H. (1981). Carbohydrate craving in obese people: Suppression by treatments affecting serotoninergic transmission. *Internal Journal of Eating Disorders, 1,* 2-11.

Wurtman, J. J., Wurtman, R. J., Mark, S., Tsay, R., Gilbert, W., & Growdon, J. (1985). d-Fenfluramine selectively suppresses carbohydrate snacking by obese subjects. *International Journal of Eating Disorders, 4,* 89-99.

Wurtman, R. J., & Wurtman, J. J. (1989). Carbohydrates and depression. *Scientific American, 260,* January, 68-75.

Wurtman, R. J., & Wurtman, J. J. (1996). Brain serotonin, carbohydrate craving, obesity and depression. *Advances in Experimental Medicine and Biology,* 398, 35-41.

Yeary, J. (1987). The use of Overeaters Anonymous in the treatment of eating disorders. *Journal of Psychoactive Drugs, 19,* 303-309.

Young, S. N. (1986). The effect on aggression and mood of altering tryptophan levels. *Nutrition Reviews, 44*(Suppl.), 112-122.

Young, S. N. (1993). The use of diet and dietary components in the study of factors controlling affect in humans: A review. *Journal of Psychiatry and Neuroscience, 18,* 235-244.

Medicinal Foods:
Cross-Cultural Perspectives

Chu-Huang Chen, MD, PhD
Devin C. Volding, MSW

SUMMARY. Knowledge of medicinal herbs and food products and the use of plants for healing date back to many ancient civilizations. Today the medicinal use of plants and foods, which is based, in part, from the knowledge of trial and error use over thousands of years in various cultures, has become incorporated into virtually all human societies. In fact, some foods and herbs have shown contemporary medicinal promise and value for their potential health promoting and protective effects. In this paper we review the literature on the medicinal value of green tea, soybean, garlic, ginger root, and *Gingko biloba,* and provide an overview of ginseng, echinacea, and St. John's wort. *[Article copies available for a fee from The Haworth Document Delivery Service: 1-800-342-9678. E-mail address: getinfo@ haworthpressinc.com <Website: http://www.haworthpressinc.com>]*

KEYWORDS. Medicinal foods, nutritional supplements, herbs, cross-cultural

INTRODUCTION

Perhaps we will never know how early humans discovered the medicinal uses of various foods. Throughout history, though, by

Chu-Huang Chen and Devin C. Volding are affiliated with the Department of Medicine/Section of Atherosclerosis, Baylor College of Medicine, Houston, TX.

Address correspondence to: Chu-Huang Chen, MD, PhD, Baylor College of Medicine, 6565 Fannin, M.S. A-601, Houston, TX 77030.

[Haworth co-indexing entry note]: "Medicinal Foods: Cross-Cultural Perspectives." Chen, Chu-Huang, and Devin C. Volding. Co-published simultaneously in *Drugs & Society* (The Haworth Press, Inc.) Vol. 15, No. 1/2, 1999, pp. 49-64; and: *Food as a Drug* (ed: Walker S. Carlos Poston II, and C. Keith Haddock) The Haworth Press, Inc., 2000, pp. 49-64. Single or multiple copies of this article are available for a fee from The Haworth Document Delivery Service [1-800-342-9678, 9:00 a.m. - 5:00 p.m. (EST). E-mail address: getinfo@ haworthpressinc.com].

© 2000 by The Haworth Press, Inc. All rights reserved.

necessity humans developed a dependent relationship with their environment for nutritional sustenance and medicinal remedies, and therefore endeavored to understand the secrets of nature. Because of this, it may be speculated that the search for such foods was driven by the urge to produce the curative and restorative means of treating illness and injury. Success ultimately was accomplished by trial and error. Knowledge of medicinal herbs and the use of plants for healing date back to ancient civilizations. In fact, discovery of a preserved grave site in Iraq provides archaeological evidence that Neanderthal man employed such healing knowledge some 60,000 years ago (Jones, 1996b).

Knowledge of medicinal herbs in China dates back approximately four or five thousand years and is attributed to the legendary emperor and sage, Sheng Nung, the "Divine Plowman," who compiled one of the first 'Herbals.' Legend suggests he collected and tasted hundreds of plants through numerous field and mountain trips in an effort to find therapeutic remedies for his people. His work and experiences were later recorded by an anonymous scribe in approximately 101 B.C. in the book *Sheng Nung Ben Cao Chien* (Shen-Nung Pen-Ts'ao Ching), or *The Herbal Classic of the Divine Plowman*, which formed the basis of Chinese herb medicine (Huang, 1993). Similar stories have been told in other cultures. Eventually these theories and practices of the medicinal uses of plants gradually spread to India, Mesopotamia, Persia, Egypt and the Eastern Mediterranean, Greece, Europe, and North America, whereupon some became compiled into 'Herbals' (Jones, 1996a).

In Mesopotamia around 2500 B.C., for example, the Sumarians are believed to have compiled their first 'Herbal' of medicinal plants. Similarly, thereafter, the medicinal qualities of plants were compiled and codified in Egypt approximately 1500 B.C. in a classic compilation of herbs, *Ebers Papyrus*. The Roman equivalent, *Historia Naturalis,* which is attributed to Pliny, likewise codified the medicinal qualities of plants (Bolton et al., 1982). In Greece around 320 B.C., Theophrastus, a pupil of Aristotle, compiled a similar work, *Inquiry into Plants* (Bolton et al., 1982). These works culminated in the first century A.D., in the work *De Materia Medica* written by Dioscorides, a Roman surgeon. Through his travels with the Roman army, he collected hundreds of medicinal plants and chronicled their medical uses.

This work remained influential and established a "standard" for herbals lasting approximately until the 15th century A.D.

More recently, North American Indians developed herbal remedies generally derived from plants in their quest to provide cures for illness and injury. One of the first such reported cures, the use of tree bark and tree leaves for scurvy, is believed to have occurred in Canada approximately 1535 A.D. (Chandler, Freeman, & Hooper, 1979). Today the medicinal use of plants, which is based, in part, from the knowledge of trial and error use over thousands of years in various cultures, has become incorporated into virtually all human cultures. Some notable herbs, in fact, have shown contemporary medicinal promise and value for their potential health promoting and protective effects. Examples of these include garlic, green tea, soybean, and *Gingko biloba,* dating back thousands of years to Asian cultures and used in traditional Chinese medicine; and, ginger root, native to India and used for centuries. In this paper we review the literature on the medicinal value of green tea, soybean, garlic, ginger root, *Gingko biloba,* and provide an overview of ginseng, echinacea, and St. John's wort. At this time we do not recommend the use of these herbal medicinals to replace conventional medical treatments.

MEDICINAL FOODS

Green Tea

Early man's consumption of tea appears to have begun some 4000 years ago in Asian cultures. In fact, the history of tea as a beverage is traced by the Chinese to approximately 3000 B.C. during the rule of Emperor Sheng Nung, and later recorded in about 350 B.C. in the Chinese wordbook, *Erh Yu* (Weisburger, 1997). Eventually, the tradition of tea consumption extended to Japanese culture around the 6th century, then throughout what is now Indonesia, India, and Europe. Tea is a product of the plant *Camellia sinensis.* It is widely consumed throughout the world in three forms: black (78%), green (20%) and oolong tea (2%) (Jankun et al., 1997). The prevalence of tea consumption is so great, it is considered the second most consumed beverage today, following the consumption of water (Weisburger, 1997).

Tea consumption is believed to have cancer prevention effects. These effects are believed to result from the tumor inhibitory activity of (−) epigallocatechin-3-gallate (EGCG) and (−) epicatechin-3-gallate (ECG), and green tea polyphenol (GTP), the main constituents of tea extracts. Tumor inhibitory activities have been demonstrated in in vitro investigations, animal models and some human studies. An example of this inhibitory activity is demonstrated in the work of Liao et al. (1995). Results indicate an intraperitoneal injection of EGCG inhibited the growth and reduced the size of induced human prostate tumors and human breast cancers in nude mice. The researchers conclude there may be a relationship between high consumption of green tea and the low incidence of prostate and breast cancers in some Asian countries. Additionally, Katiyar et al. (1997) demonstrate a similar protective effect. Specifically, GTP provided protection against induction and subsequent progression of squamous cell carcinomas in experimental protocols in mice. Topical application of polyphenol (6 mg/animal) resulted in significant protection against skin tumor promotion in terms of tumor incidence (32-60%), multiplicity (49-63%) and tumor volume/mouse (73-90%) at 20 weeks. These results suggest green tea polyphenol may afford protection against skin cancer risk in mice. Similar results have been demonstrated in some human studies. For example, Ji et al. (1996), in a retrospective study investigating 1124 patients with newly diagnosed stomach cancers and 1451 frequency matched population controls, found green tea consumption significantly decreased the risk of stomach cancer at both cardia and distal sites in men and women equally.

Tea consumption is also suggestive of preventive effects against cardiovascular diseases. These effects are likely to result from the anti-cholesterolemic activity of the tea extract. The association of green and black tea consumption with reduced blood serum cholesterol levels has been demonstrated in numerous animal models and human studies. Vinson and Dabbagh (1998), for example, found that green and black tea, compared to controls, provided significant improvement in the plasma lipid profile of hamsters. This improvement, the authors conclude, resulted from both hypolipemic and antioxidant mechanisms of the tea extract. Similar reductions in risk factors for heart disease have been demonstrated in human studies. In a retrospective study with 2062 Japanese men, Kono et al. (1996) found reductions in blood levels of total cholesterol, low-density lipoprotein cholesterol and very low-density lipoprotein cholesterol. In that investigation, high-density lipoprotein and triglyceride levels were unrelated to green tea consumption. Moreover, Imai and Nakachi (1995) found similar reductions of blood lipid profiles, combined with an increased proportion in high-density lipoprotein, in 1371 Japanese men aged over 40. These results suggest that green tea may act protectively against cardiovascular disease. Conversely, Princen et al. (1998), in a randomized, placebo-controlled study of 64 smokers during a 4-week period, found tea consumption (6 cups per day) had no effect on plasma lipids and LDL oxidation.

Soybean

Soybean products have held a prominent role in Asian cultures for centuries, both as a nutritional source and medicinal remedy. Today, while soybean products remain a nutritional staple to many Asian cultures, they are increasingly consumed throughout the world for their reported medicinal value. Soybean products, typically consumed in a variety of traditional soyfood products, are categorized into two groups: nonfermented and fermented soy products. Traditional non-fermented soyfoods include fresh green soybeans, whole dry soybeans, soy nuts, soy sprouts, wholefat soy flour, soymilk and soymilk products, tofu, okara and yuba. Traditional fermented soyfoods include tempeh, miso, soy sauces, natto and fermented tofu and soymilk products (Globitz, 1995).

Soybean products, increasingly recognized as having potential positive health promoting effects, have shown medicinal promise in the treatment and prevention of cancer and cardiovascular disease as well. Specifically, the protective effect is believed to be mediated by the isoflavone genistein, a constituent of soybean products, which contains a number of anti-carcinogens and is considered an anti-proliferative compound. Genistein is believed to modify or suppress abnormal cell growth, and thus potentially inhibit cell proliferation. For example, Messina et al. (1994), in a review investigating the consumption of soy products and cancer, found evidence of protective effects for cancer risk. Genistein suppressed the growth of a wide range of cultured cancer cells, and provided protective effects in 65% of the animal studies reviewed. The epidemiological data suggest only certain nonfermented soy products, e.g., soymilk and tofu, offered similar protection, or none at all. No consistent pattern was found with the fermented soy products investigated, such as miso. Furthermore, Barnes (1995), in a review of in vitro and animal models of cancer reported that genistein inhibited the proliferation of cultured human tumor cell lines and also reduced incidence and risk of cancer in two-thirds of the animal studies under review. Likewise, Hawrylewicz et al. (1995) reported that genistein appeared to inhibit a variety of tumors in various tissues. These studies suggest an inhibitory effect of soybean products on abnormal cell growth in various models through the antiproliferative mechanism of genistein.

Soyfoods also are believed to provide hypocholesterolemic protective effects against cardiovascular disease. These effects allegedly arise from the inhibiting action of genistein on cholesterol absorption or bile acid reabsorption, or both. Potter (1996) suggests consumption of soy protein or various extracts of soy, or both, is associated with an increase in low-density lipoprotein receptor activity in both animals and humans; hence, increased amounts of low-density lipoprotein will be absorbed in the liver. As such, soy protein or various soy extracts may exert direct beneficial cardiovascular effects and decelerate atherosclerotic progression. Furthermore, Anderson et al. (1995), in a meta-analysis of 38 controlled clinical trials investigating the effects of soy protein consumption (47 g per day) on serum lipid concentrations in humans, found consistent hypolipidemic effects as a result of soy protein consumption. These results indicate ingestion of soy protein was associated with decreases in total cholesterol (23.2 mg per deciliter, or 9.3%), low-density lipoprotein cholesterol (21.7 mg per deciliter, or 12.9%), and triglycerides (13.3 mg per deciliter, or 10.5%) with a nonsignificant increase in high-density lipoprotein cholesterol (2.4%). In summary, soy food products appear to have some protective effects against cardiovascular disease.

Garlic

Garlic, *Allium sativum,* has a long history of use for medicinal purposes dating back thousands of years to ancient Hebrew, Babylonian, Greek and Roman, and Chinese and Japanese civilizations (Bolton et al., 1982). The Egyptians believed garlic's medicinal power to be useful in treating various illnesses. Likewise, Hippocrates, Galen and Aristophanes recommended garlic for many ailments ranging from dog and snake bites, scorpion stings, asthma, madness, convulsions, tumors, consumption, gastrointestinal disorders, to its use as a diuretic (Bolton et al., 1982). Similarly, the use of garlic as a "cure-all" was employed in medieval times during the great plague. In Chinese and Japanese cultures garlic has been used medicinally for thousands of years, primarily for its cardiovascular effects in the treatment of hypertension. Garlic cloves, crushed or intact, have been used in cuisines throughout many cultures since ancient times, both for its flavor and its antiseptic potentials. In the 19th century, garlic's antiseptic effect was confirmed by the great French biologist Louis Pasteur. This therapeutic effect was extensively practiced during World War I when garlic juice, mixed with water, was used to treat wound infections of French, British, and Russian soldiers (Donaldson, 1998).

Garlic reportedly has numerous potential health promoting effects including cardiovascular protection, anti-bacterial and anti-cancer activities. The multiple beneficial cardiovascular effects of garlic include reducing total serum cholesterol levels, lowering blood pressure, and possibly acting as a blood thinner and reducing clot formations by inhibiting platelet aggregation. In a meta-analysis of controlled human trials investigating the effect of garlic to reduce hypercholesterolemia, Warshafsky et al. (1993) found that garlic (one-half to one clove per day) decreased total serum cholesterol levels by about 9% in the studied groups. Steiner et al. (1996) reported similar hypocholesterolemic effects of aged garlic extract (7.2 g per day) in a double-blind crossover study of moderately hypercholesterolemic men. Reductions of total serum cholesterol by 7.0% and low-density lipoprotein cholesterol by 4.6% were reported. In addition, systolic and diastolic blood pressure was reduced by 5.5%. Bordia et al. (1998), in a study investigating in vitro effects of garlic oil on platelet aggregation and eicosanoid metabolism, found positive inhibitory activity of garlic oil on platelet aggregation. Specifically, garlic oil inhibits thromboxane formation and platelet aggregation induced by several platelet agonists. Likewise, Harenberg et al. (1988) reported inhibitory effects of dried garlic consumption on several cardiovascular parameters, e.g., blood coagulation, fibrinolysis, platelet aggregation, serum cholesterol levels, and blood pressure, in 20 hyperlipoproteinemic patients over four weeks. Reductions in fibrinogen and fibrinopeptide A (10%), total cholesterol levels (10%), and systolic and diastolic blood pressure were reported. In addition, an increase (10%) in streptokinase activated plaminogen and fibrinopeptide B beta 15-42 also occurred.

Garlic also is believed to demonstrate numerous immune-stimulating properties, including anti-bacterial, fungicidal, and fungistatic activities. These functions are believed to be attributed to allicin, a main constituent of garlic, which may also play a role in tumor inhibition (Key et al., 1997).

Ginger Root

Ginger root, *Zingiber officinale,* indigenous to India, has been instrumental in cooking for its seasoning qualities and food preservative effects, and also healing for centuries throughout many cultures. Likewise, ginger root has been used in Asian cultures for thousands of years as a food additive for seasoning, food preservative to prevent spoilage, and for numerous medicinal purposes, including treating digestive disorders. Chinese historical records suggest that ginger root was compiled by Sheng Nung approximately 3000 B.C. Ginger, reportedly, was recommended as a medicinal tool for various ailments ranging from colds, fever, chills, tetanus, leprosy, motion sickness and nausea, to the treatment of digestive disorders (Donaldson, 1998). In fact, historical records indicate Chinese sailors chewed ginger root to prevent sea sickness. Today, in part as a result of historical traditions, many Asian dishes are flavored with ginger, because it is considered to aid digestion and possibly act as an antidote to food poisoning. The ancient Greeks are believed to have employed ginger as a medicinal aid in digestion. After meals, they wrapped ginger in bread to palliate the symptoms of indigestion; today, this custom has evolved into gingerbread, a widely consumed food.

Ginger is widely employed as a remedy for treating nausea and motion sickness for its possible anti-inflammatory, antinauseant, and antispasmodic properties. Al-Yahya et al. (1989) demonstrated that ginger extract (500 mg/kg orally) exhibited cytoprotective and anti-ulcerogenic activity against induced gastric lesions in albino rats. The ginger extract significantly reduced the formation of gastric ulcers and inhibited gastric lesions in these rats. Ginger also has shown medicinal promise in reducing nausea associated with motion sickness in some human studies. In a study comparing the effects of ginger versus dimenhydrinate and placebo in 36 undergraduate men and women with high susceptibility to motion sickness, Mowrey and Clayson (1982) found powdered ginger to be more effective than either dimenhydrinate or placebo in reducing the effects of motion sickness and gastrointestinal distress in blindfolded subjects tilted in a rotating chair. Conversely, Stewart et al. (1991), who investigated the protective effect of ginger root against motion sickness in twenty-eight subjects by rotating them in a chair just short of vomiting, found that ginger root provided no anti-motion sickness effect. In summary, the relationship of ginger root and motion sickness remains clouded.

Ginger also is believed to have anti-inflammatory properties and may possibly reduce inflammation and inflammatory symptoms associated with some types of arthritis. Sharma et al. (1994) reported that ginger oil effectively suppressed inflammation and swelling of paws and joints in experimental animals. Srivastava and Mustafa (1992) reported similar findings in their investigation examining the effects of ginger in 56 patients with rheumatism and musculoskeletal disorders, in which ginger provided relief of joint pain and swelling as well as muscular discomfort.

Ginkgo Biloba

The Ginkgo tree, *Ginkgo biloba,* has existed in China for millions of years. It can be traced to the Carboniferous Period, some 230,000 years ago (Pang et al., 1996). The Ginkgo tree has been part of traditional Chinese medicine for thousands of years. Ancient Chinese 'Herbals' make reference to the medicinal effects of the *Ginkgo biloba* leaves for treating the heart and lungs (Pang et al., 1996). While the leaves of the Ginkgo tree are considered the main medicinal resource, knowledge of *Ginkgo biloba*'s edible fruit and their valuable medicinal properties is considered unique to China. Historically, throughout Chinese culture, *Ginkgo biloba* seeds were used as a remedy for treating various ailments ranging from cancer, venereal disease, asthma, respiratory ailments, impaired hearing, to decreased sexual energy (Donaldson, 1998). Likewise, *Ginkgo biloba* has been cultivated for centuries in Japanese culture and employed for its medicinal value. In the 18th century, the Ginkgo tree was introduced to Europe, though initially as a decorative tree, and later North America.

Today *Ginkgo biloba* extract (GBE) remains one of the most widely prescribed herbs in Europe, where it is typically used for alleviating various symptoms associated with a vast array of cognitive deficits, ranging from memory impairment to dementia. The major effects indicated for Ginkgo leaves' extracts include increased blood flow with consequent improvement of memory, claudication, and tinnitus. The main extracts isolated from Ginkgo leaves are mainly flavonoids and terpene lactones. The flavonoid action is believed to reduce capillary permeability and reduce tissue injury, while the terpene lactones (ginkgolides) are believed to inhibit platelet aggregation through their antagonist activity towards the platelet-activating-factor receptor, thereby improving circulatory flow. Improvement of short-term memory resulting from the administration of GBE has been reported in the literature. For example, results from several human trials demonstrate the ability of GBE to improve mental information processing speed and short-term memory (Allain et al., 1993; Rai et al., 1991). These results provide some evidence of GBE's potential beneficial effects on memory abilities. Additionally, *Ginkgo biloba* extract (EGb 761) has been found to palliate cognitive deficits in mildly to severely demented outpatients with Alzheimer's disease in a placebo-controlled, double-blind, 52 week randomized study (Le Bars et al., 1997). When evaluated at 6 and 12 months, the EGb 761 (120 mg per day) group scored better in cognitive performance and social functions, compared with the placebo group. Therefore, EGb 761 appears to have provided cognitive-protective effects in stabilizing the cognitive deterioration of patients with Alzheimer's disease.

GBE is also believed to be useful in treating symptoms of tinnitus. For instance, Meyer (1986) found that GBE supplementation improved conditions of tinnitus in all cases in a multicenter, randomized, double-blind placebo-controlled study of 103 tinnitus outpatients during a 13-month period.

OTHER WIDELY USED HERBS

Although many herbs are not typically classified or consumed as a food per se, certain herbs are widely used for various therapeutic beliefs. Some of these herbs, e.g., ginseng, *Echinacea purpurea,* and St. John's wort, are briefly discussed here.

Ginseng

Ginseng, *Panax ginseng,* specifically considered the panacea of Chinese pharmacology for more than 2,000 years, has been used for centuries throughout many Asian cultures. Earliest evidence for its medicinal use dates back over four thousand years in the Chinese 'Herbal' *Pen-Ts'ao,* compiled approximately 3000 B.C. The knowledge of the medicinal qualities of ginseng later spread to Europe and the United States, whereupon it became a "cure-all" remedy for many ills. Today ginseng is widely consumed and believed to exhibit numerous health promoting properties and effects ranging from the prevention and treatment of aging, anemia, hyper- and hypotension, diabetes, insomnia, muscle weakness, and gastritis, to providing general stress relief (Dubick, 1983). The potential health promoting properties and effects of ginseng, though yet unsubstantiated, are currently receiving scientific investigation.

Echinacea

Echinacea, *Echinacea purpurea* and *Echinacea angustifolia,* a native of North America, was originally employed by the North American Plains Indians as a remedy to treat wounds, insect bites, stings and snake bites (Donaldson, 1998). Echinacea is widely used for its potential immune-stimulating properties in the prevention and treatment of common colds and flu, and other various infections. In vitro data has demonstrated echinacea's ability to enhance cellular immune function (See et al. 1997). Similar findings have been demonstrated in some human studies. For example, Melchart et al. (1994), in a review of 26 reported clinical tests involving echinacea, report that echinacea appeared to exert general immune-stimulation effects. More recently, however, Melchart et al. (1998), in a randomized double-blind, placebo-controlled trial investigating the protective effect of echinacea root extracts on prevention of upper respiratory tract infections in 302 volunteers, found that echinacea provided no prophylactic effect. However, the authors speculate that echinacea products may provide a 10-20% relative risk reduction.

St. John's Wort

The medicinal use of St. John's wort, *Hypericum perforatum,* dates back to the first century A.D. in Greek civilization and is believed to be attributed to Galen and Dioscorides (Donaldson, 1998), where it was commonly prescribed and employed for its wound healing properties. Today, St. John's wort extract is primarily used for its mood regulatory, antidepressant effects, in palliating depressive symptomatology. Research suggests St. John's wort extract plays a significant role in ameliorating symptoms of depression. Moreover, findings from a recent metaanalysis and overview of clinical trials suggest St. John's wort extract performed significantly better than placebo and was similarly effective as standard antidepressants, and also exhibited fewer side effects than their antidepressant counterparts (Linde et al., 1996). St. John's wort extract also is touted for its potential antiviral properties, including possible anti-tumor and antibiotic activities (Hudson et al., 1991).

DISCUSSION

Medicinal foods have gained in popularity over the past few years and are currently experiencing remarkable worldwide growth. This growth extends beyond some traditional countries such as Taiwan, Japan, and China, where medicinal food uses have an illustrious history, to many countries, including Germany, France, and the United States. Today millions of people are consuming medicinal foods to treat illness, potentially without appropriate professional advice. Miller (Johnston, 1997) indicates estimates of medicinal food use in the United States approach 33% of the population. Similar prevalence rates exist for other countries. Overall worldwide sales for herbal medicinals have become a multi-billion dollar a year market, growing approximately 20% each year.

In light of this recent surge in the use of medicinal foods, consumers, foremost, should be aware of the potential limitation of effects and risk of side effects involved with any self-medication treatment regimen bordering outside mainstream medical practices. There exists a likelihood for potentially harmful adverse effects associated with these treatment regimens, especially in light of the fact that many are in need of further scientific investigation. For instance, Miller (1998) reports on numerous drug-herb interactions currently. Echinacea, for example, if used beyond 8 weeks, is believed to cause hepatotoxicity. Therefore, if used concomitantly with certain other hepatoxic medications, e.g., anabolic steroids, amiodarone, methotrexate, and ketoconazole, it potentially can have deleterious health effects. Certain other herbal medicinals, e.g., *Ginkgo biloba,* garlic, ginger and ginseng, are believed to alter circulatory functioning. As such, certain anticoagulant medications, if used concurrently, could potentially be problematic. In some instances, however, only relatively minor adverse side effects are indicated with the use of herbal medicinals. Some of these adverse side effects range from minor gastrointestinal upset (*Ginkgo biloba*), headaches (ginseng and *Ginkgo biloba*), to photosensitivity

(St. John's wort extract). Long-term or incorrect use of ginkgo may cause excessive bleeding. One case report, for example, revealed bleeding in the head with long-term use of ginkgo extract (120 mg daily for two years). Fortunately, the patient was cured by removal of the blood and discontinuation of ginkgo (Rowin & Lewis, 1996). Another report showed bleeding in the eye in a patient who took both ginkgo extract (40 mg, twice a day) and aspirin daily. The bleeding stopped after discontinuation of gingko (Rosenblatt & Mindel, 1997).

As a result of the current state of knowledge surrounding herbal medicinals, we are not recommending the use of herbal medicinals to replace regular medical treatments. Long-term prospective clinical investigations are needed to provide clarification regarding the safety and efficacy of herbal medicinals and delineate potential risk-benefit analyses so that definitive relationships regarding mechanism of action, potential side effects and potential and known drug-herb interactions might be better understood. Although research has elucidated many potential health promoting effects of some herbal medicinals, numerous scientific questions remain unanswered. These questions are due, in part, to a lack of long-term controlled clinical trials. The preponderance of studies are either short-term or are based on animal or cell in vitro data. Because of this, extrapolating from current research results to human use is, in some cases, premature and unwarranted. As such, the use of herbal medicinals must be carried out with great caution.

REFERENCES

Al-Yahya, M. A., Rafatullah, S., Mossa, J. S., Ageel, A. M., Parmar, N. S., & Triq, M. (1989). Gastroprotective activity of ginger *Zingiber officinale* Rosc., in albino rats. *American Journal of Chinese Medicine*, 17, 51-56.

Allain, H., Raoul, P., Lieury, A., LeCoz, F., Gandon, J. M., & d'Arbigny, P. (1993). Effect of two doses of *Ginkgo biloba* extract (EGb 761) on the dual-coding test in elderly subjects. *Clinical Therapeutics*, 15, 549-558.

Anderson, J. W., Johnstone, B. M., & Cook-Newell, M. E. (1995). Meta-analysis of the effects of soy protein intake or blood serum lipids. *The New England Journal of Medicine*, 333, 276-282.

Barnes, S. (1995). Effect of genistein on in vitro and in vivo models of cancer. *Journal of Nutrition*, 125 (3, Suppl), 777S-783S.

Bolton, S., Null, G., & Troetel, W. M. (1982). The medical uses of garlic–Fact and fiction. *American Pharmacy*, NS22, 40-43.

Bordia, A., Verma, S. K., & Srivastava, K. C. (1998). Effect of garlic (*Allium sati-*

vum) on blood lipids, blood sugars, fibrinogen and fibrinolytic activity in patients with coronary artery disease. *Prostaglandins Leukotrienes and Essential Fatty Acids,* 58 (4), 257-263.

Bowman, W. C. (1979). Drugs ancient and modern. *Scottish Medical Journal,* 24, 131-140.

Chandler, R. F., Freeman, L., & Hooper, S. N. (1979). Herbal remedies of the Maritime Indians. *Journal of Ethnopharmacology,* 1, 49-68.

Donaldson, K. (1998). Introduction to the healing herbs. *ORL-Head and Neck Nursing,* 16 (3), 9-16.

Dubick, M. A. (1986). Historical perspectives on the use of herbal preparations to promote health. *Journal of Nutrition,* 116, 1348-1354.

Globitz, P. (1995). Traditional soyfoods: Processing and products. *Journal of Nutrition,* 125, 570S-572S.

Harenberg, J., Giese, C., & Zimmermann, R. (1988). Effect of dried garlic on blood coagulation, fibrinolysis, platelet aggregation and serum cholesterol levels in patients with hyperlipoproteinemia. *Atherosclerosis,* 74 (3), 247-249.

Hawrylewicz, E. J., Zapata, J. J., & Blair, W. H. (1995). Soy and experimental cancer: Animal studies. *Journal of Nutrition,* 125, 698S-708S.

Huang, K. C. (1993). *The Pharmacology of Chinese Medicinal Herbs.* Boca Raton, FL: CRC Press.

Hudson, J. B., Lopez-Bazzocchi, I., & Towers, G. H. N. (1991). Antiviral activities of Hypericin. *Antiviral Research,* 15, 101-112.

Imai, K., & Nakachi, K. (1995). Cross sectional study of effects of drinking green tea on cardiovascular and liver disease. *British Medical Journal,* 310, 693-696.

Jankun, J., Selman, S. H., Swiercz, R., & Skrzypczak-Jankun, E. (1997). Why drinking green tea could prevent cancer. *Nature,* 387 (6633), 561.

Ji, B. T., Chow, W. H., Yang, G., McLaughlin, J. K., Gao, R. N., Shu, X. O., Jin, F., Fraumeni, J. F., Jr., & Gao, Y. T. (1996). The influence of cigarette smoking, alcohol, and green tea consumption on the risk of carcinoma of the cardia and distal stomach in Shanghai, China. *Cancer,* 77, 2449-2457.

Johnston, B. A. (1997). One-third of nation's adults use herbal remedies. *Herbalgram,* 40, 49.

Jones, F. A. (1996a). Herbs–Useful plants. Their role in history and today. *European Journal of Gastroenterology & Hepatology,* 8, 1227-1231.

Jones, F. A. (1996b). Herbs: Useful plants. *Journal of the Royal Society of Medicine,* 89, 717-719.

Katiyar, S. K., Mohan, R. R., Agarwal, R., & Mukhtar, H. (1997). Protection against induction of mouse skin papillomas with low and high risk of conversion to malignancy by green tea polyphenols. *Carcinogenesis,* 18, 497-502.

Key, T. J., Silcocks, P. B., Davey, G. K., Appleby, P. N., & Bishop, D. T. (1997). A case-controlled study of diet and prostate cancer. *British Journal of Cancer,* 76 (5):678-687.

Kono, S., Shinchi, K., Wakabayashi, K., Honjo, S., Todoroki, I., Sakurai, Y., Imanishi, K., Nishikawa, H., Ogawa, S., & Katsurada, M. (1996). Relation of green tea consumption to serum lipids and lipoproteins in Japanese men. *Journal of Epidemiology,* 6, 128-133.

Le Bars, P. L., Katz, N. M., Berman, N., Itil, T. M., Freedman, A. M., & Schatzberg, A. F. (1997). A placebo-controlled, double-blind, randomized trial of an extract of *Ginkgo biloba* for dementia. *Journal of the American Medical Association, 278,* 1327-1332.

Liao, S., Umekita, Y., Guo, J., Kokontis, J. M., & Hiipakka, R. A. (1995). Growth inhibition and regression of human prostate and breast tumors in athymic mice by tea epigallocatechin gallate. *Cancer Letters, 96,* 239-243.

Linde, K., Ramirez, G., Mulrow, C. D., Pauls, A., Weidenhammer, W., & Melchart, D. (1996). St. John's wort for depression–An overview and meta-analysis of randomized clinical trials. *British Medical Journal, 313,* 253-258.

Melchart, D., Linde, K., Worku, F., Bauer, R., & Wagner, H. (1994). Immunomodulation with echinacea–A systematic review of controlled clinical trials. *Phytomedicine, 1,* 245-254.

Melchart, D., Walther, E., Linde, K., Brandmaier, R., & Lersch, C. (1998). Echinacea root extracts for the prevention of upper respiratory tract infections: A double-blind, placebo-controlled randomized trial. *Archives of Family Medicine, 7*(6), 541-545.

Messina, M. J., Persky, V., Setchell, K. D., & Barnes, S. (1994). Soy intake and cancer risk: A review of the in vitro and in vivo data. *Nutrition and Cancer, 21,* 113-131.

Meyer, B. (1986). Multicenter randomized double-blind drug vs. placebo study of the treatment of tinnitus with *Ginkgo biloba* extract. *La Presse Médicale, 15,* 1562-1564.

Miller, L. G. (1998). Herbal medicinals: Selected clinical considerations focusing on known or potential drug-herb interactions. *Archives of Internal Medicine, 158* (20), 2200-2211.

Mowrey, D. B., & Clayson, D. E. (1982). Motion sickness, ginger, and psychophysics. *The Lancet, 1,* 655-657.

Pang, Z., Pang, F., & He, S. (1996). *Ginkgo biloba L.*: History, current status, and future prospects. *The Journal of Alternative and Complementary Medicine, 2,* 359-363.

Potter, S. M. (1996). Soy protein and serum lipids. *Current Opinion In Lipidology, 7,* 260-264.

Princen, M. G., van Duyvenvoorde, W., Buytenhek, R., Blonk, C., Tijburg, L. B. M., Langius, J. A. E., Meinders, A. E., & Pijl, H. (1998). No effect of consumption of green tea and black tea on plasma lipid and antioxidant levels and on LDL oxidation in smokers. *Arteriosclerosis Thrombular & Vascular Biology, 18,* 833-841.

Rai, G. S., Shovlin, C., & Wesnes, K. A. (1991). A double-blind, placebo controlled study of *Ginkgo biloba* extract ('tanakan') in elderly outpatients with mild to moderate memory impairment. *Current Medical Research and Opinion, 12,* 350-355.

Rosenblatt, M., & Mindel, J. (1997). Spontaneous hyphema associated with ingestion of *Ginkgo biloba* extract. *New England Journal of Medicine, 336,* 1108.

Rowin, J., & Lewis S. L. (1996). Spontaneous bilateral subdural hematomas associated with chronic *Ginkgo biloba* ingestion. *Neurology, 46,* 1775-1777.

See, D. M., Broumand, N., Sahl, L., & Tilles, J. G. (1997). In vitro effects of echinacea and ginseng on natural killer and antibody-dependent cell cytotoxicity in healthy subjects and chronic fatigue syndrome or acquired immunodeficiency syndrome patients. *Immunopharmacology*, 35(3), 229-235.

Sharma, J. N., Srivastava, K. C., & Gan, E. K. (1994). Suppressive effects of eugenol and ginger oil on arthritic rats. *Pharmacology*, 49, 314-318.

Srivastava, K. C., & Mustafa, T. (1992). Ginger (*Zingiber officinale*) in rheumatism and musculoskeletal disorders. *Medical Hypotheses*, 39, 342-348.

Steiner, M., Khan, A. H., Holbert, D., & Lin, R. I. (1996). A double-blind crossover study in moderately hypercholesterolemic men that compared the effect of aged garlic extract and placebo administration on blood lipids. *The American Journal of Clinical Nutrition*, 64, 866-870.

Stewart, J. J., Wood, M. J., Wood, C. D., & Mims, M. E. (1991). Effects of ginger on motion sickness susceptibility and gastric function. *Pharmacology*, 42(2), 111-120.

Vinson, J. A. & Dabbagh, Y. A. (1998). Effect of green and black tea supplementation on lipids, lipid oxidation and fibrinogen in the hamster: Mechanisms for the epidemiological benefits of tea drinking. *FEBS Letters*, 433(1-2), 44-46.

Warshafsky, S., Kamer, R. S., & Sivak, S. L. (1993). Effect of garlic on total serum cholesterol. A meta-analysis. *Annals of Internal Medicine*, 119 (7, Pt. 1), 599-605.

Weisburger, J. H. (1997). Tea and health: A historical perspective. *Cancer Letters*, 114, 315-317.

Legal and Regulatory Perspectives on Dietary Supplements and Foods

Walker S. Carlos Poston II, PhD
Laurie Fan, MBA
Rich Rakowski, PharmD
Martin Ericsson, MD, PhD
Christopher C. Bunn, MS
John P. Foreyt, PhD

SUMMARY. Dietary supplements, including vitamins, minerals, tissue extracts, amino acids, protein products, and herbal preparations to enhance health or prevent disease are used by nearly fifty percent of the U.S. population. They are a 12+ billion dollar market. The purpose of this review is to provide background information on the prevalence and uses of dietary supplements, the legislation pertaining to dietary supplements, including the Dietary Supplement Health and Education Act of

---

Walker S. Carlos Poston II is Assistant Professor, Department of Psychology, University of Missouri-Kansas City and Co-Director of Behavioral Cardiology Research, Mid America Heart Institute, St. Luke's Hospital, Kansas City, MO. Laurie Fan and Rich Rakowski are affiliated with BioNutritional Encyclopedia, Inc. Martin Ericsson is affiliated with the Baylor College of Medicine and The Swedish National Social Insurance Hospital, Nynäshamn, Sweden. Christopher C. Bunn is affiliated with the University of Texas, Houston Health Science Center. John P. Foreyt is affiliated with the Baylor College of Medicine.

Address correspondence to: Walker S. Carlos Poston II, PhD, Co-Director of Behavioral Cardiology, Mid America Heart Institute, St. Luke's Hospital, 5319 Holmes, Kansas City, MO 64110 (E-mail: postonwa@umk.edu).

The authors wish to acknowledge that this work was partially supported by a Minority Scientist Development Award from the American Heart Association and with funds contributed by the AHA, Puerto Rico Affiliate.

[Haworth co-indexing entry note]: "Legal and Regulatory Perspectives on Dietary Supplements and Foods." Poston, Walker S. Carlos, II et al. Co-published simultaneously in *Drugs & Society* (The Haworth Press, Inc.) Vol. 15, No. 1/2, 1999, pp. 65-85; and: *Food as a Drug* (ed: Walker S. Carlos Poston II, and C. Keith Haddock) The Haworth Press, Inc., 2000, pp. 65-85. Single or multiple copies of this article are available for a fee from The Haworth Document Delivery Service [1-800-342-9678, 9:00 a.m. - 5:00 p.m. (EST). E-mail address: getinfo@haworthpressinc.com].

© 2000 by The Haworth Press, Inc. All rights reserved. 65

1994 and the Food and Drug Modernization Act of 1997, and to summarize their impact on the quality, safety, and marketing of dietary supplements. Four case examples, white willow bark, sassafras, ephedrine, and St. John's Wort are presented. Finally, the problems associated with the current regulatory standards and the potential changes that could improve the quality, standardization, and safety are discussed. *[Article copies available for a fee from The Haworth Document Delivery Service: 1-800-342-9678. E-mail address: getinfo@haworthpressinc.com <Website: http://www.haworthpressinc.com>]*

KEYWORDS. Dietary supplements, regulation, Dietary Supplement Health and Education Act, FDA, drugs, herbs

INTRODUCTION

What are dietary or nutritional supplements and why is it important to discuss them? The current widespread use of dietary supplements in the U.S. has important implications for individuals, health care providers, and the Food and Drug Administration (FDA) because many of these supplements are being used and promoted as aids or treatments for various health conditions. More importantly, there is a lack of safety and efficacy data for most of these supplements, creating a significant public health dilemma.

The purpose of this review is to provide background information on dietary supplements, how extensively they are used, and their economic costs. We then review legislation pertaining to dietary supplements, including the Dietary Supplement Health and Education Act of 1994 and the Food and Drug Modernization Act of 1997, and summarize their impact on the use and sale of dietary supplements, using four case examples. Finally, we will outline the dangers associated with the current regulatory standards and present potential changes that could improve the quality, standardization, and safety of dietary supplements.

PREVALENCE OF DIETARY/NUTRITIONAL SUPPLEMENT USE IN THE U.S.

Dietary supplements include vitamins (used at recommended daily allowances or megadoses exceeding ten times the recommended daily allowance), minerals, tissue extracts (e.g., glandular products), amino acids and protein products, and herbal preparations (i.e., crude plant drugs utilized for the treatment of disease states, often chronic, to attain or maintain improved health) (Eliason, Kruger, Mark, & Rasmann, 1997; Tyler, 1987; 1994). The Dietary Supplement Health and Education Act of 1994 defines a dietary supplement as a product intended to supplement the diet that contains one or more of the following ingredients: (1) a vitamin; (2) a mineral; (3) an herb or other botanical; (4) an amino acid; (5) a dietary substance for use to supplement the diet by increasing the total dietary intake; or (6) a concentrate, metabolite, constituent, extract, or combination of any of the previously described ingredients. In addition, the Act goes on to specify that dietary supplements are not represented for use as conventional foods. Thus, the FDA considers dietary supplements more like foods and not drugs (Durden Beltz & Doering, 1993; Eliason, Myszkowski, Marbella, & Rasmann, 1996).

Dietary supplements typically have been used for the purpose of correcting dietary deficiencies, enhancing health and/or performance (i.e., ergogenic aids), and preventing and/or treating disease. The last two uses appear to be the most important reasons that people report for taking dietary supplements (De Smet, 1993). Many individuals turn to supplements which promise increased energy. For example, more than 100 companies market "ergogenic aids" and "energy enhancers," with over 300 products containing more than 230 ingredients, including wheat germ, bee pollen, Ma Huang (ephedra), guarana (caffeine), amino acids, ginseng, and other herbs and mineral combinations which have little or no scientific validation of efficacy (Herbert & Barrett, 1994). When customers accessed a new computer-based nutrition supplement teaching program at 400 stores of a major health food store chain, "fatigue" was the most asked about symptom and total sales of ergogenic products exceeded $204 million in 1996 (McCarthy, 1997).

Similarly, when Sobal and colleagues (Pally, Sobal, & Muncie, 1984: Sobal, Muncie, & Guyther, 1986) surveyed several hundred patients in urban and rural family health centers, they found that most patients reported taking supplements to increase their energy and reduce fatigue, ensure good nutrition, prevent illness, and improve their strength and ability to deal with stress. Data from two more recent surveys of nearly 400 patients provide similar results. For example,

Eliason et al. (1997) found that 84.3% of the patients that responded to their survey reported taking supplements to increase their wellness and prevent disease. The rest, 15.7%, reported taking them to treat perceived health problems.

In another study by Eliason and colleagues (1996), patients were asked about their specific reasons for taking supplements. Patients most frequently reported the benefits of supplements to be improved energy/nutrition and enhanced immune function/disease prevention (52.4%). The remaining perceived benefits reported (47.6%) fell within the category of disease intervention. These perceived benefits included treatment of musculoskeletal disorders, women's health concerns, psychological/central nervous system concerns, hematological, dermatological, gastrointestinal, and cardiovascular problems, pain, and weight loss.

While the exact prevalence of dietary supplement use in the U.S. is not known, several studies provide a picture of ubiquitous use, consistent with the public's increased use of alternative methods of health care (Eisenberg, Kessler, Foster, Norlock, Calkins, & Delbanco, 1993). Depending on the survey population, estimates of dietary supplement use range from 31% to 66% (Sobal et al., 1986). For example, a survey of 128 patients in an urban family health center found that 31% currently used supplements, while a survey by the same investigators of rural patients found 54% used supplements (Pally et al., 1984; Sobal et al., 1986).

In a larger survey using data from the 1987 National Health Interview Survey (NHIS) of 22,080 adults aged 18-99, 51.1% of the respondents reported consuming a dietary supplement over the past year, with 23.1% taking them on a daily basis (Subar & Block, 1990). Multivitamins were the most commonly consumed supplements. More recently, Eliason and colleagues (1996) surveyed 200 consecutive patients at a family practice clinic and found that 52% had used supplements during the previous year. Of that group, 32% took 1 supplement and 20% took from 2 to 13 different supplements. Of the supplements taken, 84% were multivitamins and minerals while the rest were herbal compounds, amino acids, proteins, and other supplements.

Who is the typical consumer of dietary supplements? While it is difficult to develop an accurate profile due to the lack of large, population-based investigations, several studies provide some insight. Eliason et al. (1996) reported that family practice clinic patients with a college education took more supplements than those who only had graduated from high-school. In their second study of health food store consumers, Eliason et al. (1997) found the typical customer was a middle-aged (40-49) Caucasian female who was educated beyond high school. The most generalizable study (Subar & Block, 1990), using 22,080 participants in the NHIS study, found that middle-aged Caucasian women were the ones most likely to use dietary supplements. Among all participants, those most likely to use supplements were older (in all gender and ethnicity categories), had more education (i.e., at least high school and some college), and had higher incomes (i.e., were more likely to be employed in "white-collar" professions).

Given the extensive use of supplements, what is their economic impact? While it is difficult to calculate an exact figure on sales associated with supplement use, several investigators have developed estimates of their economic significance. Eisenberg and colleagues (1993) found that respondents in their survey of alternative medicine consumption spent an average of $431 per person per year for dietary supplements, yielding a national projection of nearly $2 billion dollars. With regard to herbal preparations alone, the market was estimated to be as large as $1.2 to 1.5 billion dollars in U.S. sales (Ernst, 1998; Tyler, 1996) and $11.9 to 12.5 billion worldwide (in U.S. dollars), with at least half of that spent in Europe (Anonymous, 1997; De Smet & Brouwers, 1997).

Taken together, these data suggest that dietary supplement use is widespread in the U.S. and that most people use them to improve their health and energy and to prevent or treat diseases. In addition, consumers are willing to spend substantial amounts of money on dietary supplements. It is therefore understandable that there is interest and concern, both on the part of the consumer and regulatory agencies, about their quality, safety, and efficacy.

THE LEGAL STATUS OF DIETARY SUPPLEMENTS AND THE ROLE OF THE FDA

While several laws play a role in the regulation of dietary supplements, the two recent primary sources for guidance are the Dietary Supplement Health and Education Act of 1994 and the Food and Drug Modernization Act of 1997. Before summarizing these Acts, it is important to review how previous legislation led to their development, i.e., to understand their current status, it is necessary to have some knowledge of laws relating to drug sales.

The first significant federal regulation of pharmaceuticals was the Food and Drug Act of 1906, which is often referred to as the "Pure" Food and Drug Act, which prohibited the interstate sales of mis-branded and adulterated foods, beverages, and drugs. This Act was the first attempt to halt the rampant fraud among food and drug producers (Tyler, 1994). In 1912 the Sherley Amendment was added by Congress, which prohibited the labeling of medicines with false therapeutic claims, after the Supreme Court ruled that the 1906 Act only prohibited false and misleading statements about the ingredients or identity of a drug and not the making of false therapeutic claims. This Act and amendment substantially reduced fraudulent practices in the pharmaceutical industry, such as misbranding and adulteration, but failed to address effectively the issues of safety and efficacy (Tyler, 1986; 1994).

In 1938, after a drug containing 72% diethylene glycol was mar-keted in the southern U.S. and was linked to over 100 deaths due to kidney failure, the Federal Food, Drug, and Cosmetic Act was passed. This legislation required that all new drugs entering interstate com-merce be proven safe, eliminated the Sherley Amendment requirement for proving intent to defraud in drug misbranding cases, and provided for safe tolerances of unavoidable toxic substances. Unfortunately, drugs that were already on the market were subject to the 1906 Act and were grandfathered, requiring no further proof of safety.

In 1962 the thalidomide tragedy occurred in Europe (the drug caused severe birth defects but was never marketed in the U.S.). In response to this tragedy, several amendments (i.e., the Drug Amend-ments of 1962) to the 1938 Act were passed that required all drugs marketed in the U.S. after 1962 be proven both safe and effective, but drugs marketed prior to 1938 were grandfathered. While this Act was the first of its kind to address these issues, it allowed many existing substances, particularly those in the dietary supplement category to bypass the requirement for safety and efficacy data (Tyler, 1986; 1994; 1996). While the FDA did not have any direct authority over dietary supplements, it was allowed to declare a substance (i.e., a drug or dietary supplement) as misbranded if an efficacy claim was made without adequate substantiation (Tyler, 1994).

Thus, prior to 1962, a dietary supplement, particularly an herbal preparation, could have been considered a drug if the manufacturer made a therapeutic claim. After 1962, when FDA required that all drug manufacturers (i.e., anyone making a therapeutic claim) submit safety and efficacy data, dietary supplement manufacturers began to market their products as foods, and FDA typically made no moves to regulate these products as long as no efficacy claims were made (Quinn Youngkin, & Israel, 1996). These early Acts led to the development of the next important legislative landmarks, the Dietary Supplement Health and Education Act of 1994 and the Food and Drug Modernization Act of 1997.

SUMMARY OF THE DIETARY SUPPLEMENT HEALTH AND EDUCATION ACT OF 1994

The Dietary Supplement Health and Education Act of 1994 defines dietary supplements broadly (as stated earlier) as any product intended to supplement the diet that contains one or more of the following ingredients: (1) a vitamin; (2) a mineral; (3) an herb or other botanical; (4) an amino acid; (5) a dietary substance for use to supplement the diet by increasing the total dietary intake; or (6) a concentrate, metabolite, constituent, extract, or combination of any of the previously described ingredients. The Act does not specify any safety or efficacy requirements, but it does require that the Federal Government bear the "burden of proof" in demonstrating that a supplement is unsafe or adulterated. Under the Act, a dietary supplement is adulterated if it contains an ingredient that (1) presents a "significant or unreasonable risk or illness or injury" under the conditions of recommended use or suggested labeling or under ordinary conditions of use if no such recommendations are specified; (2) is new and for which there is inadequate information to provide reasonable assurance that it does not present a significant or unreasonable health risk; or (3) poses an imminent public health or safety hazard.

However, like any other foods, it is the manufacturer's responsibility to ensure that its products are safe and properly labeled prior to marketing. The Act requires manufacturers to use a standardized label which provides complete information about product content, including ingredients, amount per serving, information on calories, calories from fat, carbohydrate, protein, sugar, etc., when present at significant levels, information on ingredients that do not have a recommended daily intake, and, if the product contains a proprietary blend, the total amount of the blend and the identity of the constituents. The label must be accompanied by a disclaimer stating that the FDA has not reviewed the supplement and that it is not to be used as a drug (Quinn Youngkin & Israel, 1996).

The Act also provides that retail outlets may make available "third-party" materials to help inform consumers about any health-related benefits of dietary supplements. These materials include articles, book chapters, scientific abstracts, or other third-party publications. These provisions stipulate that the information must not be false or misleading; cannot promote a specific supplement brand; must be displayed with other similar materials to present a balanced view; must be displayed separate from supplements; and may not have other information attached (product promotional literature, for example). Finally, the Act does not allow health or therapeutic claims on the labels of dietary supplements. A statement describing the product's role in affecting the structure or function in humans is allowed, as is accompanying literature that presents a balanced view of the scientific literature.

In summary, while this legislation clarifies what a dietary supplement is and how it should be labeled, it does not require the producer to demonstrate that the supplement is safe or effective. In fact, it puts the burden for proving lack of safety on the FDA, a situation that has added to the confusion about supplement benefits and the lack of standardization and development in supplement research in the U.S. (Tyler, 1996). Additionally, while it grants FDA the authority to establish manufacturing regulations governing the preparation, packing, and holding of dietary supplements under conditions that ensure their safety, no such regulations ensuring quality control and standardization have yet been developed.

SUMMARY OF THE FOOD AND DRUG MODERNIZATION ACT OF 1997

The Food and Drug Modernization Act of 1997 is divided into five sections or titles and is aimed at improving the regulation of drugs, devices, and foods. Titles I and II deal with the regulation of drugs and devices and Titles IV and V are the general provisions and effective dates. Title III (Improving the regulation of food) is most pertinent to dietary supplements. In short, this Act authorizes the FDA to make regulations regarding health and disease prevention claims and nutrient descriptors. Thus, the Act authorizes the use of disease prevention or health claims in food labeling based on published authoritative statements (i.e., a balanced representation of the scientific literature which may include a bibliography of the literature) from a scientific body of the U.S. government, e.g., the National Institutes of Health (NIH), Centers for Disease Control and Prevention (CDC), or the National Academy of Sciences (NAS). The statements must be about the relationship between a nutrient and a disease or health-related condition, they must be stated in a manner that accurately represents the statement, and they must enable the public to understand the significance of the information. Finally, a claim submitted under Title III of this Act may be made until the FDA issues a regulation modifying or prohibiting the claim. Thus, as in the Dietary Supplement Health and Education Act of 1994, the FDA has the burden for proving lack of safety or mislabeling.

SYNTHESIS OF THE LEGISLATION

The distinction between dietary supplements and drugs, and food in some cases, is not always clear. For example, the FDA defines a drug as any substance recognized in the official U.S. Pharmacopoeia (or National Formulary) for internal or external use, or as substances or a mixture of substances intended to be used for the cure, mitigation, or prevention of disease of either man or other animals (FDC, 1938). In addition, drugs, when taken by a living organism, may modify one or more of its functions (Thomas, 1989). It is clear that many dietary supplements, and even some foods, can alter or modify physiological functions (Christensen, 1996; Tyler, 1994).

In addition, many dietary supplements and some foods are used to treat or prevent diseases. Several dietary supplements have been studied extensively for the treatment of various diseases ranging from osteoarthritis to depression and some macronutrients have been found to play an important role in mood (Christensen, 1996; Tyler, 1994). The primary distinction, at least from the perspective of the FDA, is with respect to how health claims are made. Both Acts outline requirements for what kind of claims can be made about a substance, stating that health/disease or therapeutic claims can only be made if a new drug application (NDA) is filed and premarket approval is granted. Otherwise, supplement (and food) marketers must restrict themselves to claims about how the products affect the structure or function in humans or, in the case of foods, they can make health claims if they are based on published authoritative statements from a national scientific body. This exception for foods could potentially propel some supplement manufacturers to market their products as foods, and clearly, some products that have been defined as dietary supplements also could be defined as foods (e.g., protein and amino acid products).

THE IMPACT OF LEGISLATION ON THE QUALITY, SAFETY, AND USE OF DIETARY SUPPLEMENTS

What is the impact of these Acts on improving the quality, safety, and use of dietary supplements? Four case examples of dietary supplements are reviewed to provide insight into the benefits and problems inherent in the current legislation as it pertains to dietary substances. First, we review the appropriate application and safety and efficacy for each supplement. Then we provide an analysis of the impact of the legislation given the background safety and efficacy data.

Example 1–Probably Safe but Ineffective. The Case of White Willow Bark: White willow bark comes from the white willow tree, *Salix alba,* which is commonly found in Europe, Asia, and North America. The first recorded descriptions of the therapeutic benefits of white willow bark extracts were made by Hippocrates. Native Americans used the white willow bark to treat fever, diarrhea, and sore throat. White willow bark contains salicin (a precursor of aspirin). White willow bark is commonly used as a tea, using 2-3 grams of finely chopped or coarsely powdered bark, which is added to cold water and heated until boiling. After 5 minutes of boiling, the liquid is poured through a strainer. A cup of tea is drunk 3 to 4 times a day. Side-effects are not expected given the amount of salicylate extracted from the white willow bark. On the other hand, the small amounts of salicin in white willow bark tea make its use as a painkiller or fever medication impractical. It would take approximately 14 g of willow bark prepared in 10 cups of tea to yield a single dose of salicin (1 g), the average amount needed to reduce pain or fever (Tyler, 1994). Thus it is unlikely to have a therapeutic benefit.

Example 2–Unsafe and Ineffective. The Case of Sassafras: Widely used as an ergogenic tonic, sassafras, from the root bark of *Sassafras officinalis,* has historically been used as an performance enhancer, based on the belief that it can purify the blood. There are currently no data to support ergogenic health claims and sassafras has no significant therapeutic utility (Tyler, 1994). In fact, sassafras extract has been shown to be carcinogenic in animal models and the FDA has prohibited the use of sassafras-based products as food additives and flavorings (Kapadia et al., 1978; Segelman, Segelman, Karliner, & Sofia, 1976; Tyler, 1994; 1996).

Example 3–Probably Unsafe but Effective? The Case of Ephedra: Ephedrine, a stimulant anorexiant usually combined with caffeine and/ or aspirin, has been used as a weight loss agent for many years. There have been several randomized, double-blind, placebo-controlled trials of ephedrine. Few of these studies followed participants or maintained blinded conditions longer than one year (Astrup, Breum, Toubro et al., 1992; Daly, Krieger, Dulloo et al., 1993; Toubro, Astrup, Breum et al., 1993). In general, ephedrine and caffeine (EC) produced greater weight loss than dietary restriction alone, although the placebo-subtracted weight loss is modest, i.e., the placebo subtracted weight loss was 3.4 kg (Astrup, Breum, Toubro et al., 1992; Toubro, Astrup, Breum et al., 1993). In one study (Toubro, Astrup, Breum et al., 1993), the double-blind was broken between weeks 26 and 50 and patients were continued in an open-label trial. Treated patients (N = 99 from the treatment and placebo groups in the first 24 weeks) lost an additional average of 1.1 kg after 50 weeks.

There are few data on long-term EC administration (Atkinson, Blank, Loper et al., 1995). One study examined extended administration of EC combined with aspirin for 7 months in 24 obese patients and then extended unblinded treatment for another 19 months (i.e., 26 months total), but only 6 patients participated in this extension (Daly, Krieger, Dullo et al., 1993). After 8 weeks, the placebo subtracted weight loss was 1.9 kg and after 5 months, the remaining patients lost an average of 5.2 kg. While substantial safety concerns have not been raised in short-term trials, side-effects including nervousness, insomnia, and increased heart rate and blood pressure have been reported. In sensitive individuals, or in the case of overdose, ephedrine may cause stroke, heart attack, chest pain, seizures, insomnia, nausea, fatigue, dizziness, palpitations, convulsions, breathing problems, high blood pressure, and death (Cetaruk & Aaron, 1994). Some fatalities have been reported in healthy individuals (Anonymous, 1996). The ephedrine-caffeine combination is not approved for the treatment of obesity and the FDA recently has expressed serious concerns about the safety of ephedrine.

Example 4–Probably Safe and Effective. The Case of St. John's Wort/Hypericin: St. John's Wort extract (*Hypericum perforatum*) is a perennial, shrubby plant commonly found in Europe and the U.S. that historically has been used to elevate mood and treat depression. There are many active components in the extract including hypericin, pseudohypericin, carotenoids, flavonoids, xanthones, and others. It is not known which chemical is most important for its antidepressant effects. St. John's Wort has been studied extensively for its antidepressant effects, primarily in Germany where it is a prescription medication.

Numerous small, randomized, double-blind clinical trials have produced similar and consistent results in mildly to moderately depressed patients (Ernst, 1995; Harrer & Sommer, 1994; Hänsgen, Vesper, & Ploch, 1994; Hübner, Lande, & Podzuweit, 1994; Witte, Harrer, Kaptan et al., 1995). For example, Harrer and Sommer (1994) conducted a double-blind, placebo-controlled study with 105 outpatients diagnosed with depression. Patients received hypericin (300 mg, 3 times per day) or a placebo for four weeks. Hypericin-treated patients demonstrated significant reductions in depressive symptoms at both 2 and 4 weeks compared to patients receiving placebo. Similarly, Witte and colleagues (1995) conducted a multi-center, placebo-controlled, double-blind study with 97 outpatients diagnosed with depression. Patients received hypericin (100 mg to 120 mg, twice per day) or placebo. Patients taking the hypericin experienced a statistically significant reduction in depressive symptoms. The investigators reported that the St. John's Wort preparation was well tolerated, no side-effects were reported, and the response rate (70%) was excellent.

A meta-analytic review (Linde, Ramirez, Mulrow et al., 1996) covering 23 randomized and blinded trials with 1,757 patients, over 2-12 weeks of treatment with dosages varying from 300-900 mg/day demonstrated that St. John's Wort extract was consistently and significantly more effective than placebo and similarly effective when compared to standard antidepressant medications. In addition, St. John's Wort extract appears to have fewer side effects than standard antidepressants (Vorbach, Annoldt, & Hubner, 1997; Wheatley, 1997). Finally, the majority of controlled studies reported the absence of significant adverse effects or toxicity. In a large safety and side-effects monitoring study of more than 3,000 patients, undesired side-effects were reported by 2.4% of patients and 1.5% discontinued treatment (Woelk, Burkhard, & Grünwald, 1994).

SYNTHESIS AND IMPLICATIONS OF THE CASE STUDIES

White willow bark and sassafras provide examples of supplements that are generally ineffective and yet are still available on the market. While white willow bark appears to be benign and at worst, a waste of money for the consumer, sassafras has demonstrated carcinogenicity, but is still touted in some sources as a health tonic (Tyler, 1994). As noted earlier, the FDA was concerned enough about the safety of sassafras to ban its use as a flavoring, but it is still available as a supplement, thus highlighting a problem with the reactive nature of the current legislation. Because FDA has the burden of proof require-ment, it is unlikely that sassafras can be removed from the market unless enough problems are reported or if its manufacturers/distribu-tors make false health claims.

Ephedrine and St. John's Wort present interesting examples of di-etary supplements that have been used to treat specific health prob-lems (i.e., obesity and depression) and have reasonable efficacy data. St. John's Wort also has good safety and toxicity studies, but the safety of ephedrine is in question (Anonymous, 1996; Anonymous, 1997; Quinn Youngkin, & Israel, 1996). In fact, since 1994, the FDA has received over 800 reports of ephedrine-related adverse events ranging from insomnia and nervousness to seizures, stroke, and death (Anony-mous, 1997). While these reports propelled the FDA to develop regu-lations to address the concerns, including substantial marketing and labeling changes (e.g., no marketing of products containing more than 8 milligrams (mg) of ephedrine, no labeling that would suggest ingest-ing more than 8 mg in a six-hour period or 24 mg per day, warnings about health risks associated with excessive use, and more extensive general warning labels), they illustrate a major weakness in the current system–the lack of proactivity. In other words, a dietary supplement must begin to demonstrate enough safety problems that it "catches the eye" of the FDA before any significant action can be taken.

St. John's Wort highlights another problem with current legislation. St. John's Wort appears to be a safe and effective treatment for depression, at least in short term studies. In addition, it is a prescription medication in Germany. But in the U.S. it has virtually no status in the medical community even though it might provide a reasonable treatment alternative to standard tricyclic antidepressants and selective serotonin reuptake inhibitors (SSRIs) with fewer side effects. In essence, because St. John's Wort is a natural product, and therefore not patentable, it is an unlikely candidate for drug companies to pursue and establish safety and efficacy data to meet FDA requirements (Tyler, 1994; 1996).

In addition, because it is classified as a dietary supplement, the manufacturers have no financial incentive to pursue FDA approval, which would make it more acceptable to the American medical community. Finally, because it does not have to meet FDA requirements for safety and efficacy, manufacturers have no incentive to ensure adequate quality control (i.e., Do all St. John's Wort supplements have the amounts of hypericin that produced antidepressant effects in German clinical trials?). Remember that neither the Dietary Supplement Health and Education Act of 1994 nor the Food and Drug Modernization Act of 1997 require evidence of quality control, purity, safety, or efficacy for dietary supplements and both put the burden of proving lack of purity and/or safety on the FDA. Because the FDA is one small agency, it is unlikely that it can adequately police a multibillion dollar industry with over 600 manufacturers producing more that 4000 products (Dietary Supplement Health and Education Act of 1994).

SHORTCOMINGS OF THE CURRENT REGULATIONS AND POTENTIAL SOLUTIONS

The Potential Dangers of Dietary Supplements

The above cases highlight several important limitations in the current regulatory approach to dietary supplements. For example, none of the prior legislation addresses the issue of supplement standardization and quality control in a proactive manner. While it is true that the FDA can pursue a manufacturer for adulteration, the burden of proof is on the FDA. Several investigators have noted that supplement quality control is a significant problem in the U.S., with many marketed products not containing any or the necessary amount of the compound of interest (Tyler, 1987). Linked to this issue of standardization and quality control is the problem of misidentified herbs and compounds in commercial and consumer-prepared dietary supplements which can result in cases of toxicity and fatality. For example, herbal preparations and the relative concentrations of the active compounds may vary greatly depending on the part of the plant used (e.g., the stem, roots, leaves), the developmental stage of the plant when it was harvested, where it was grown, the conditions of its harvesting and storage, and the methods of extraction (Cetaruk & Aaron, 1994). The only way to know the true concentration, purity, and make-up (i.e., the constituent compounds) is for manufacturers to perform assays, which is rarely done due to lack of governmental pressure (Quinn Youngkin & Israel, 1996).

The current legislation also does not require any proof of safety/nontoxicity or efficacy unless the FDA is made aware of potential mislabeling, i.e., the manufacturer makes an unsubstantiated health claim. This situation promulgates the lack of research on dietary supplement safety and efficacy and contributes to inadequate consumer information. For example, Eliason and colleagues (1997) found that fifty of the products that their sample reported using have been reported in the literature as causing toxic reactions. Even a reasonably safe and effective supplement like St. John's Wort can have potential pharmacological interactions that could lead to serious health problems (Miller, 1998). St. John's Wort extract is hypothesized to be a SSRI or a monoamine oxidase inhibitor (MAOI) (Miller, 1998; Neary & Bu, 1999; Raffa, 1998). Because MAOIs can cause severe hypertension if foods are eaten that contain tyramine, it is possible that St. John's Wort extract may cause a similar problem (Clark, Brater, & Johnson, 1988; Suzuki, Katsumata, Oya, Bladt, & Wagner, 1984). Therefore, certain medications, such as those contraindicated while taking MAOIs, probably should be avoided while taking St. John's Wort.

St. John's Wort also may have interaction problems with other serotonergic drugs, causing "serotonin syndrome" if taken with drugs that release or prevent the reuptake of serotonin. Serotonin syndrome is a potentially life threatening complication characterized by varied degrees of cognitive, autonomic, and neuromuscular dysfunction, often due to the combination of MAOIs and serotonin enhancing drugs, such as SSRIs (Hilton, Maradit, & Moller, 1997; Ivanusa, Hecimovic, & Demarin, 1997; Mills, 1997). If this is the case for a dietary supplement with adequate research, what is the likelihood that there could be similar or worse problems that are yet unknown for hundreds of dietary supplements and combinations of supplements that have minimal or virtually no safety or toxicity research? It is reasonable to suggest that most supplements have not been adequately studied and their safety, efficacy, and drug interactions are largely unknown (D'Arcy, 1993; Eliason et al., 1997; Ernst, 1998; Miller, 1998).

Related to the above issue, it is important to note that consumer studies suggest that patients tend to get most of their information about dietary supplements from the media and other non-scientific sources (Eliason et al., 1996; Tyler, 1986). More disturbingly, many patients, over one-third in one study (Eliason et al., 1996), do not tell their physicians or other health care providers that they are taking supplements. In addition, many consumers use supplements for health conditions or preventive purposes and not for the health problems they reserve for their physician (Eisenberg et al., 1993). This situation increases the possibility of patients improperly dosing themselves on supplements or taking ones that may negatively interact with medications that they are receiving from their physician.

A final shortcoming of the current system is that the regulations provide no inducements or incentives to dietary supplement manufacturers to engage in research and report safety and efficacy data. Because manufacturers can market their products with claims that are not disease-based, but suggest enhancements of normal structure and function, they can sell products that may be just as pharmacologically potent and hazardous as any synthetic drug (Cetaruk & Aaron, 1994). In defense of manufacturers, the situation is complicated by the fact that natural products are difficult, if not impossible, to patent (i.e., they do not meet the novelty criteria required for patents because many have been used for hundreds of years). In addition, the process of developing a new drug and filing a new drug application (NDA) with the FDA is a time-consuming and expensive process that may exceed 12 years and 230 million dollars (Tyler, 1994).

Potential Solutions for the Future

What is needed for satisfactory, reasonable, and modest reform? At the most basic level, established quality standards are needed for dietary supplements. Consumers need to be assured that what they are taking is indeed the intended supplement. Manufacturers should be required, or at least strongly encouraged, to meet pharmaceutical production standards with regard to supplement identity, purity, composition, and dosage (Tyler, 1994; 1996). With herbal preparations in particular, standard and consistent nomenclatures need to be developed. For example, Tyler (1994) suggests that Latin binomials be preferred over common or folklore names.

On a larger and more complicated scale, dietary supplement safety, efficacy, and claims must be reexamined (Tyler, 1994). The current approach in the U.S. is to not require any safety or efficacy data and to permit no health claims. As discussed earlier, the "no claims" approach does not preclude manufacturers from "wordsmithing" labels so that they meet the regulations while still presenting the product in an unbalanced manner. In addition, manufacturers can mislabel their product with a health claim under the premise that the FDA may not find out until after they have already made a significant profit since premarket safety and efficacy research is not necessary and current regulations require the FDA to demonstrate that the product is mislabeled.

There are alternatives to the U.S. model, but their acceptability in the current litigious climate is questionable. For example, Canadian health officials have struggled with a proposal to designate some products that are labeled as dietary supplements in the U.S. as "Folklore Medicines" (Tyler, 1994). While the whole of this proposal was not adopted, some commonly used herbs were allowed to be marketed with limited health/disease claims based on their traditional uses. A drawback to this approach is that it still allows for inaccurate and fraudulent claims and does not promote safety and efficacy research.

The model that might be most useful is the one that predominates in Germany. The German government permits health claims based on "reasonable" proof of safety and efficacy, and is based on the German Federal Health Agency's Commission E, whose members established a system for evaluating supplement safety and efficacy (Tyler, 1996). Tyler (1994) has suggested that it might be appropriate for the FDA to adopt the German Commission E system, which is now a series of published monographs that are being translated into English. As Tyler (1994) points out, precedent exists because many drugs now approved in the U.S. were first approved in other countries. On the other hand, this also presents the dilemma of requiring one set of standards for supplements and a more rigorous, difficult, and costly standard for synthetic drugs. Unfortunately, there is no way around this problem because supplement manufacturers cannot patent their products, thus negating the possibility that they will pursue an NDA.

De Smet and Brouwer (1997) suggest that the principle of proportionality should apply to supplements. This principle suggests that premarketing requirements for supplements with good quality control, a wide margin of safety, and limited claims for minor indications or concerns should need only minimal regulatory oversight. Those substances that are recommended for serious disorders and which may have significant or major side-effects would require that same safety and efficacy data needed for synthetic drugs. Unfortunately, this still does not address the patentability issue for manufacturers. None of these solutions is optimal, nor do they address all of the potential pitfalls or double-standards that might develop between supplements and synthetic drugs.

CONCLUSION

There are no clear and simple solutions for regulating dietary supplements. None of the potential solutions are completely satisfactory and the most promising option, that used by the United German Republic with the Guidance of the Commision E, would create a problematic double-standard between supplements and synthetic drugs. Nevertheless, the status quo is worse than any of the potential solutions because it results in a misinformed and ignorant public, very little research on safety and efficacy in the U.S., and it allows the FDA to respond only after potential problems have been identified.

This situation is partly a function of our current health paradigm and its artificial distinction between supplements and drugs, based on where and how the product was created. In order to truly profit from the potential health benefits of natural products, including dietary supplements and foods, we will have to broaden our thinking about concepts of health, wellness, disease, treatment, and cure. If we do not, then the future of this promising area is bleak (Tyler, 1987). Consumers and physicians will remain misinformed and continue to use supplements inappropriately, other countries will take the lead in research and development, and potentially significant medications and treatments may never be discovered.

REFERENCES

Anonymous (1996). Adverse events associated with ephedrine-containing products–Texas, December 1993-September 1995. *MMWR, 45,* 689-693.

Anonymous (1997). FDA proposes constraints on ephedrine dietary supplements. *American Journal of Health Systems Pharmacy, 54,* 1578.

Anonymous (1997). FDA and Pharmanex clash over dietary supplement. *Nature Biotechnology, 15,* 100.

Astrup, A., Breum, L., Toubro, S., Hein, P., & Quaade, F. (1992). The effect and safety of an ephedrine/caffeine compound compared to ephedrine, caffeine and placebo in obese subjects on an energy restricted diet. A double blind trial. *International Journal of Obesity and Related Metabolic Disorders, 16,* 269-277.

Atkinson, R. L., Blank, R. C., Loper, J. F., Schumacher, D., & Lutes, R. (1995). Combined drug treatment of obesity. *Obesity Research, 3(Suppl. 4),* 497S-500S.

Barrett, S. J., & Herbert, V. (1994). *The vitamin pushers: How the "Health Food" industry is selling America a bill of goods.* New York: Prometheus Books.

Cetaruk, E. W., & Aaron, C. K. (1994). Hazards of nonprescription medicines. *Emergency Medicine Clinics of North America, 12,* 483-510.

Clark, W. G., Brater, D. C., & Johnson, A. R. (1988). *Goth's Medical Pharmacology (12th Edition)* (pp. 268-277). St. Louis, MO: The C. V. Mosby Company.

Christensen, L. (1996). *Diet-behavior relationships: Focus on depression.* Washington, D.C.: American Psychological Association.

D'Arcy, P. F. (1993). Adverse reactions and interactions with herbal medicines. Part 2–Drug interactions. *Adverse Drug Reactions and Toxicology Review, 12,* 147-162.

Daly, P. A., Krieger, D. R., Dulloo, A. G., Young, J. B., & Landsberg, L. (1993). Ephedrine, caffeine and aspirin: Safety and efficacy for treatment of human obesity. *International Journal of Obesity and Related Metabolic Disorders, 17(Suppl. 1),* S73-S78.

De Smet, P. A. G. M. (1993). An introduction to herbal pharmacoepidemiology. *Journal of Ethnopharmacology, 38,* 197-208.

De Smet, P. A. G. M., & Brouwers, R. B. J. (1997). Pharmacokinetic evaluation of herbal remedies: Basic introduction, applicability, current status, and regulatory needs. *Clinical Pharmacokinetics, 32,* 427-436.

Dietary Supplement Health and Education Act of 1994 (Public Law 103-417: 103rd Congress, 2d Session Senate) (pp. 1-49). Washington D.C.: Report 103-410.

Eisenberg, D. M., Kessler, R. C., Foster, C., Norlock, F. E., Calkins, D. R., & Delbanco, T. L. (1993). Unconventional medicine in the United States: Prevalence, costs, and patterns of use. *New England Journal of Medicine, 328,* 246-252.

Eliason, B. C., Kruger, J., Mark, D., & Rasmann, D. N. (1997). Dietary supplement users: Demographics, product use, and medical system interaction. *Journal of the American Board of Family Practice, 10,* 265-271.

Eliason, B. C., Myszkowski, J., Marabella, A., Rasmann, D. N. (1996). Use of dietary supplements by patients in a family practice clinic. *Journal of the American Board of Family Practice, 9,* 249-253.

Ernst, E. (1995). St. John's Wort, an anti-depressant? A systematic, criteria-based review. *Phytomedicine, 2,* 67-71.

Ernst, E. (1998). Harmless herbs? A review of the recent literature. *American Journal of Medicine, 104*, 170-178.

Food, Drug, and Cosmetic Act, as Amended, §201 (h)(g), 21 U.S.C., §321 (h) (g).

Food and Drug Modernization Act of 1997 (143 Congressional Record, H8482 (October, 1997).

Hänsgen, K.-D., Vesper, J., & Ploch, M. (1994). Multicenter double-blind study examining the antidepressant effectiveness of the hypericum extract LI 160. *Journal of Geriatric Psychiatry and Neurology, 7(Suppl. 1)*, S15-S18.

Harrer, G., & Sommer, H. (1994). Treatment of mild/moderate depressions with Hypericum. *Phytomedicine, 1*, 3-8.

Hilton, S. E., Maradit, H., Moller, H. J. (1997). Serotonin syndrome and drug combinations: Focus on MAOI and RIMA. *European Archives of Psychiatry & Clinical Neuroscience, 247*, 113-119.

Hübner, W.-D., Lande, S., & Podzuweit, H. (1994). Hypericum treatment of mild depressions with somatic symptoms. *Journal of Geriatric Psychiatry and Neurology, 7(Suppl. 1)*, S12-S14.

Ivanusa, Z., Hecimovic, H., & Demarin, V. (1997). Serotonin syndrome. *Neuropsychiatry, Neuropsychology, & Behavioral Neurology, 10*, 209-212.

Kapadia, G. J., Chung, E. B., Ghosh, B., Shukla, Y. N., Basak, S. P., Morton, J. F., & Pradhan, S. N. (1978). Carcinogenicity of some folk medicinal herbs in rats. *Journal of the National Cancer Institute, 60*, 683-686.

Linde, K., Ramirez, G., Mulrow, C. D., Pauls, A., Weidenhammer, W., & Melchart, D. (1996). St John's Wort for depression–An overview and meta-analysis of randomized clinical trials. *British Medical Journal, 313*, 253-258.

McCarthy, L. (1997). Report on use of the computer-based bionutritional encyclopedia. Norwalk, CT: New Paradigm Ventures, unpublished report.

Miller, L. G. (1998). Herbal medicinals: Selected clinical considerations focusing on known or potential drug-herb interactions. *Archives of Internal Medicine, 158*, 2200-2211.

Mills, K. C. (1997). Serotonin syndrome: A clinical update. *Critical Care Clinics, 13*, 763-783.

Neary, J. T., & Bu, Y. (1999). Hypericum LI 160 inhibits uptake of serotonin and norepinephrine in astrocytes. *Brain Research, 816*, 358-363.

Pally, A., Sobal, J., Muncie, H. L. Jr. (1984). Nutritional supplement utilization in an urban family practice center. *Journal of Family Practice, 18*, 249-253.

Quinn Youngkin, E., & Israel, D. S. (1996). A review and critique of common herbal alternative therapies. *Nurse Practitioner, 21*, 39-52.

Raffa, R. B. (1998). Screen of receptor and uptake-site activity of hypericin component of St. John's Wort reveals sigma receptor binding. *Life Sciences, 62*, 265-270.

Segelman, A. B., Segelman, F. P., Karliner, J., & Sofia, R. D. (1976). Sassafras and herb tea. Potential health hazards. *JAMA, 236*, 477.

Sobal, J., Muncie, H. L. Jr., Guyther, J. R. (1986). Nutritional supplements use by patients in a rural family practice. *Journal of the American College of Nutrition, 5*, 313-316.

Subar, A. F., & Block, G. (1990). Use of vitamin and mineral supplements: Demographics and amounts of nutrients consumed. The 1987 Health Interview Survey. *American Journal of Epidemiology, 132,* 1091-1101.

Suzuki, O., Katsumata, Y., Oya, M., Bladt, S., & Wagner, H. (1984). Inhibition of monoamine oxidase by hypericin. *Planta Medica, 50,* 272-274.

Thomas, C. L. (Ed.) (1989). *Taber's Cyclopedic Medical Dictionary (16th Edition).* Philadelphia, PA: F. A. Davis Company.

Toubro, S., Astrup, A. V., Breum, L., & Quaade, F. (1993). Safety and efficacy of long-term treatment with ephedrine, caffeine and an ephedrine/caffeine mixture. *International Journal of Obesity and Related Metabolic Disorders, 17(Suppl. 1),* S69-S72.

Tyler, V. (1987). Herbal medicine in America. *Planta Medica, 53,* 1-4.

Tyler, V. (1994). *Herbs of choice: The therapeutic use of phytomedicinals.* New York: Pharmaceutical Products Press.

Tyler, V. (1996). What pharmacists should know about herbal remedies. *Journal of the American Pharmaceutical Association, NS36,* 29-37.

Vorbach, E. U., Arnoldt, K. H., & Hubner, W. D. (1997). Efficacy and tolerability of St. John's Wort Extract LI 160 versus imipramine in patients with severe depressive episodes according to ICD-10. *Pharmacopsychiatry, 30(Suppl 2),* 81-85.

Wheatley, D. (1997). LI 160, an extract of St. John's Wort, versus amitriptyline in mildly to moderately depressed outpatients–A controlled 6-week clinical trial. *Pharmacopsychiatry, 30(Suppl 2),* 77-80.

Witte, V. B., Harrer, G., Kaptan, T., Podzweit, H., & Schmidt, U. (1995). [Treatment of depression with a highly concentrated hypericum preparation. A multicenter, placebo-controlled, double-blind study]. *Fortschritte Der Medizin, 113,* 404-408.

Woelk, H., Burkard, G., & Grünwald, J. (1994). Benefits and risks of the hypericum extract LI 160: Drug monitoring study with 3250 patients. *Journal of Geriatric Psychiatry and Neurology, 7(Suppl. 1),* S34-S38.

Eating Disorders and Addiction

G. Terence Wilson, PhD

SUMMARY. Eating disorders show some similar features to substance abuse and dependence, but this does not justify viewing them as an addiction. Neither tolerance nor withdrawal reactions to food have been demonstrated. Evidence for "carbohydrate craving" is lacking, and other ostensibly common features (e.g., loss of control over eating, preoccupation with food) have biobehavioral explanations that do not invoke addiction. While not an addiction, eating disorders have been reliably linked to substance abuse and dependence in clinical and community samples. However, the association is not a specific one, and the mechanisms that explain it are unknown. Independent familial transmission of eating and substance use disorders indicates that they do not derive from a single, shared etiological mechanism. Clinicians should routinely screen for substance abuse in eating disorder patients and vice versa. *[Article copies available for a fee from The Haworth Document Delivery Service: 1-800-342-9678. E-mail address: getinfo@haworthpressinc.com <Website: http:// www.haworthpressinc.com>]*

KEYWORDS. Addictions, eating disorders, carbohydrate craving, treatment

As defined by *DSM-IV*, eating disorders include anorexia nervosa, bulimia nervosa, and subthreshold variations of these two disorders, called Eating Disorders Not Otherwise Specified (EDNOS) (Ameri-

G. Terence Wilson is affiliated with Rutgers University.

Address correspondence to: G. Terence Wilson, PhD, Oscar K. Buros Professor, Rutgers The State University, Graduate School of Applied and Professional Psychology, 152 Frelinghuysen Avenue, Piscataway, NJ 08854.

[Haworth co-indexing entry note]: "Eating Disorders and Addiction." Wilson, G. Terence. Co-published simultaneously in *Drugs & Society* (The Haworth Press, Inc.) Vol. 15, No. 1/2, 1999, pp. 87-101; and: *Food as a Drug* (ed: Walker S. Carlos Poston II and C. Keith Haddock) The Haworth Press, Inc., 2000, pp. 87-101. Single or multiple copies of this article are available for a fee from The Haworth Document Delivery Service [1-800-342-9678, 9:00 a.m. - 5:00 p.m. (EST). E-mail address: getinfo@haworthpress inc.com].

© 2000 by The Haworth Press, Inc. All rights reserved.

can Psychiatric Association, 1994). Obesity is neither an eating disorder nor a psychiatric disorder. A significant minority of obese patients do, however, suffer from binge eating and have the diagnosis of Binge Eating Disorder (BED) which is an example of EDNOS. It is a widely held view among practitioners, especially substance abuse counsellors, that eating disorders are a form of addiction just as is alcohol or drug abuse and dependency. As such, eating disorders can be treated with the same type of 12-Step program that is recommended for substance abusers. The seminal assumption behind this thinking is that food is a drug. Food, either literally or functionally, can act as a drug and become abused like a drug. This assumption can be challenged on both logical and empirical grounds.

THE ADDICTION MODEL: CONCEPTUAL AND EMPIRICAL SHORTCOMINGS

Eating disorders do resemble substance abuse problems in many ways. There is loss of control (that defines binge eating); reported "craving" for food; preoccupation with thoughts about food or substance; use of food to cope with negative emotions, and often repeated failed attempts to overcome the problem. But these similarities do not make eating disorders an addiction. The following are some of the conceptual and empirical difficulties with the addiction model of eating disorders.

1. Defining characteristics of chemical dependency or addiction are tolerance, physical dependence and withdrawal. No evidence exists demonstrating that any of these phenomena occur in eating disorder patients.

2. There is no compelling evidence that people with eating disorders experience craving as a direct biochemical result of consuming a particular food to which they are sometimes said to be allergic (Bemis, 1985; Wardle, 1987). A subset of obese people are said to crave carbohydrates and snack selectively on carbohydrate-rich foods (Wurtman, 1988). Carbohydrates increase tryptophan, which, in turn, enhances the release of serotonin in the brain. Accordingly, it is claimed that food functions as a form of self-medication for regulating negative affect. The validity of this theory for eating disorders remains unproven. Indeed, the data are unsupportive. For example, Turner et al. (1991) conducted an experimental analysis of the psychological

and biological effects of a simulated carbohydrate binge in bulimia nervosa patients and matched controls. Each group consumed a 500-ml drink consisting of either 1,200 kcal of carbohydrates or an inactive placebo mixture "of negligible calorific value" on two consecutive mornings following a fast. Overall, the results showed little carbohydrate-specific effect on subjective responses. What effects there were tended to be negative. In the control subjects, ratings of hunger were significantly decreased during the 2 hours following consumption of both drinks, although the effect was greater for the carbohydrate challenge. In the bulimia nervosa patients, hunger ratings were depressed before and after consumption, with no significant difference between the carbohydrate and placebo drinks. The patients also reported greater increases in nausea after carbohydrate consumption. Ratings of mood were not improved by the consumption of the carbohydrate drink. Measures of prolactin, growth hormone, and cortisol failed to indicate any carbohydrate-medicated stimulation in either group.

There is no evidence that bulimia nervosa patients preferentially consume sugar and other carbohydrates during binge eating. When the binge eating and other eating of bulimia nervosa patients and the eating of normal controls are studied directly in the laboratory, macronutrient selection is similar for both groups. The most striking difference between the binge and non-binge meals of bulimic patients is the amount of food consumed, not its macronutrient composition. This suggests that the essential appetitive abnormality in bulimia nervosa is in the control of amount of food consumed, not in the craving for a specific macronutrient (Walsh, Kissileff, Cassidy, & Dantzioc, 1989). The same holds true for obese binge eating (Yanovski et al., 1992).

3. Food might well help to regulate affect in some people. This does not necessarily make it an addictive substance. Many activities regulate affect, from health-promoting meditation to such self-destructive behavior as cutting in parasuicidal patients.

4. Food, obviously, has important biological consequences. This truism hardly makes it an "addictive" substance. Many activities have biological effects, such as stress, exercise, sex, and sleep. Vitousek (personal communication) points out that someone who is sleep deprived will "crave" and be preoccupied with sleep. It is not because they are "addicted" to sleep, but rather that they are in an abnormal biological state that needs to be remedied (normalized) by sleep. In

like fashion, the bulimia nervosa patient is preoccupied with food not because she is addicted, but because she is food deprived as a result of excessive dietary restraint. The biological and psychological sequelae of this dietary restriction trigger binge eating (Fairburn, 1997). The appropriate treatment for the food deprived bulimia nervosa patient is to restore more normal, regular eating patterns. When this is done, both craving and binge eating typically disappear (Fairburn, Marcus, & Wilson, 1993).

Consider the following clinical case illustration. Carolyn has suffered from bulimia nervosa for 10 years. She was preoccupied with controlling her body weight and shape by rigid dieting. She skipped meals and avoided specific "forbidden foods," especially ice cream. But once or twice a week she lost control and binged. As part of her cognitive-behavioral treatment (CBT) (Fairburn et al., 1993), I encouraged her to cease dieting, eat three regular meals each day, and deliberately consume some previously "forbidden foods." Carolyn insisted that she could not eat ice cream without binge eating. She believed that ice cream per se automatically triggered loss of control over eating. I encouraged her to test this firmly held belief. I suggested an alternative explanation for her binge eating. She had binged after eating ice cream in the past because, by violating her rigid diet, guilt combined with her actual hunger to cause loss of control. (In the context of alcohol dependence, Marlatt and Gordon [1985] have described this process as an abstinence violation reaction.)

Carolyn decided that she could not trust herself to keep ice cream in her house, but did agree to make plans with her teenage daughter to go out for ice cream during the afternoon. Our goal was to change the biological and psychosocial conditions under which she ate ice cream. Instead of being hungry, she would have eaten lunch. Instead of being alone and feeling vulnerable as in the past, she would have the support and pleasure of being with her daughter, with whom she was emotionally close. Carolyn ate the ice cream, experienced no loss of control, and came away empowered by the event. The point here is that it demonstrates that loss of control (binge eating) has less to do with the nutrient properties of the specific food than the biological and psychosocial conditions under which the food is consumed.

5. Fairburn (1993) points out that patients with bulimia nervosa who binge eat are intent on limiting food intake in pursuit of weight control. Binge eating seems to follow the collapse of dietary control

and causes the individual concern that this will lead to weight gain. It is the concern about body weight and shape that is driving their dieting. There is no comparable phenomenon in substance abuse. Alcoholics do not begin drinking because they are pursuing sobriety or because they fear inebriation.

6. The addiction approach to overeating fails to discriminate among the different eating disorders and obesity, which is not a psychiatric disorder at all. Obese binge eaters differ from normal weight bulimia nervosa patients in several important respects. For example, obese binge eaters do not report the same dietary control outside of binge eating. Another important difference is that many obese binge eaters appear to have begun binge eating prior to attempting to lose weight. In individuals with bulimia nervosa, dietary restraint virtually always precedes binge eating. Thus, the binge eating of overweight persons would seem to more closely resemble the unstructured and uncontrolled consumption of substance abusers, and it would be more logical to explore possible commonalties. Overweight binge eaters commonly seek help in Overeaters Anonymous groups.

TREATMENT IMPLICATIONS

The addiction model necessarily calls for a 12-step approach to the treatment of eating disorders. In an adaptation from the treatment of substance abuse disorders, it prescribes constant dietary restraint, featuring avoidance of particular foods (e.g., white sugar), highly structured eating patterns, a sense of powerlessness, and reinforcement of a dichotomous thinking pattern (Bemis, 1985). Two points must be emphasized in this connection. First, there is an absence of any scientific evidence attesting to the clinical utility of this approach. Second, and more importantly, the prescriptions of the addiction model conflict with much of what is now known about the maintenance and modification of binge eating in bulimia nervosa (Fairburn, 1997). For example, CBT, the most effective treatment for bulimia nervosa (Wilson & Fairburn, 1998), is devoted to replacing rigid dieting with regular meals featuring flexible nutrition with no forbidden foods as illustrated in the case of Carolyn above. "Abstinence" would be counterproductive since rigid dietary restriction only serves to maintain the disorder. Simply put, if the addiction model were correct, CBT could not possibly have lasting effectiveness. This clearcut disconfirmation of a strong prediction by the addiction model is especially damaging to the approach.

Attempts to make the 12-step approach more compatible with evidence-based treatments for eating disorders have sought to reframe core principles such as abstinence from particular foods as abstention from activities such as binge eating and overexercising (Johnson & Sansone, 1993). This only blurs the distinctiveness of the 12-step approach without adding substantively to existing data-based models. More generic features of 12-step groups, such as social support, are valuable but not unique to this approach.

A fundamental tenet of Alcoholics Anonymous is the Serenity Prayer–"God, grant me the serenity to accept the things I cannot change, the courage to change the things I can, and the wisdom to know the difference." Elsewhere I have discussed how this theme applies to the treatment of eating disorders (Wilson, 1996). Body shape and weight, the core concerns of patients with eating disorders, are features of all eating disorders that cannot be changed or over which patients have only limited control. Once nutritionally sound and psychologically adaptive lifestyle changes have been made, patients need to accept whatever shape and weight these changes produce. But emphasizing a balance between acceptance and change does not mean that patients must acknowledge their powerlessness over food or turn over control to some higher power. In CBT, developing acceptance is an active process of self-affirmation or empowerment (Wilson, 1996).

COMORBIDITY OF EATING
AND SUBSTANCE ABUSE DISORDERS

Eating disorders may not be a form of substance abuse, but the two problems seem related.

Substance Abuse in Clinical and Community Samples of People with Eating Disorders

Rates of lifetime substance abuse are consistently higher in patients with anorexia nervosa and bulimia nervosa than in the general population (Braun, Sunday, & Halmi, 1994; Holderness et al., 1994; Wilson, 1993). In contrast to this consistent finding, the prevalence of substance abuse in obese binge eaters has not been reliably shown to be greater than in obese controls (Mitchell & Mussell, 1995; Yanovski et al., 1993).

It is well-known that people with more than one problem are more likely to seek treatment than those with only an eating disorder. Therefore, clinical samples may be unrepresentative subsets of people with eating disorders. The only way to establish an inherent association between the two disorders is to study representative community samples. Three major epidemiological studies have provided data suggesting that there is an association between eating and substance abuse disorders. In the first study from the U.S., an analysis of over 2,000 female twins from the Virginia population-based twin register showed a significant lifetime association between bulimia nervosa and substance abuse (Kendler et al., 1991). The second study consisted of a nonclinical, community sample in Ontario, Canada (Garfinkel et al., 1995). Thirty-one percent of people with bulimia nervosa had a lifetime history of alcohol dependence compared with only 5% of community controls. A third study from New Zealand compared the comorbidity of lifetime psychiatric disorder in a clinical sample of women with bulimia nervosa and in women with bulimia nervosa in the community with the general population base rates (Bushnell et al., 1994). Consistent with previous research, the clinical sample of bulimia nervosa patients showed much higher rates of substance abuse (44%) than women in the general population (11%). In addition, the women with bulimia nervosa in the community also showed more substance abuse (34%) than normal controls.

Two other studies, however, have yielded inconsistent data. The first, based on data from the Epidemiological Catchment Area study in the U.S., found no association between alcoholism and anorexia nervosa (Helzer & Pryzbeck, 1988). Bulimia nervosa was not assessed. The second study from England compared a community sample of 102 women with bulimia nervosa with 204 normal controls and 102 patients with another psychiatric disorder (mainly depression) (Welch & Fairburn, 1996). Bulimia nervosa cases did not differ from either of the two control groups in terms of current alcohol consumption. Nor did bulimia nervosa cases differ from the psychiatric controls in terms of their history of alcohol intake. Bulimia nervosa cases used more illicit drugs than either control group, but loss of control over drug use was very uncommon. Welch and Fairburn (1996) concluded that "the differences in drug misuse cannot be assumed to reflect impulsivity; at least some drug use was described by those with bulimia nervosa as purposeful, namely the use of amphetamines for appetite control" (p. 457). In a separate analysis of the data from this study, Welch and Fairburn (1998) reported that a higher proportion of the bulimia nervosa cases were smokers than of either comparison group. Of those smokers who had achieved a period of abstinence, bulimia nervosa cases were more likely than normal control subjects to have resumed smoking.

Is There a Specific Association Between Eating Disorders and Substance Abuse? Two sets of findings suggest that the association is not a specific one. First, in clinical samples substance abuse occurs at least as frequently among patients with other psychiatric disorders, such as anxiety disorders (Kushner, Sher, & Beitman, 1990). Based on the epidemiological data, Bushnell et al. (1994) concluded that there is not a specific association between bulimia nervosa and substance abuse disorder. Rather, "the presence of any disorder is associated with a non-specific increase in the likelihood of other psychiatric disorder" (p. 605).

Second, the evidence consistently indicates that the comorbidity of both anxiety and mood disorders with eating disorders is higher than that of substance abuse (Garfinkel et al., 1995; Laessle et al., 1989).

Are Patients with Bulimia Nervosa and Comorbid Substance Abuse a Distinctive Subgroup? It has been suggested that eating disorders patients with comorbid substance abuse are a separate subgroup who differ from patients who do not abuse alcohol or drugs. In a study of this possibility, Grilo et al. (1995) compared three groups: inpatients with and without substance, and those with substance abuse disorder only. Comprehensive assessment showed high rates of overlap in *DSM-III-R* Axis I disorders. The only difference was in terms of Axis II disorders. Inpatients with substance abuse had higher rates of Cluster B personality disorders, whereas those with no comorbid substance abuse disorder had higher rates of Cluster C personality disorders. These data provide little support for the notion of a distinctive subgroup.

A well-controlled study by Lilenfeld et al. (1997) provides more persuasive evidence for the existence of a distinctive subgroup. Rates of social phobia, conduct disorder, and both Cluster B and C personality disorders were significantly higher in bulimia nervosa patients with comorbid substance abuse than patients with bulimia nervosa only or community controls. Moreover, there were differences between the first-degree relatives of the two bulimia nervosa groups. Relatives of bulimia nervosa patients with substance abuse had higher rates of social phobia, panic disorder, substance dependence, and Cluster B personality disorders than bulimia nervosa patients without substance abuse. Lilenfeld et al. (1997) suggest that the bulimia nervosa patients with substance abuse fit the description of the so-called "multi-impulsive" subtype of bulimia nervosa that has been proposed by Lacey (1993) and Fichter et al. (1994). This would have to be confirmed in epidemiological research. However, based on their case-control community study that avoided the inherent biases of clinical samples, Welch and Fairburn (1996) concluded that women with bulimia nervosa and comorbid substance abuse "are probably heterogeneous in character, and their classification as a subgroup would therefore be premature" (p. 451).

Eating Disorders in Clinical and Community Samples of People with Substance Abuse Disorders

If eating disorders and substance abuse do occur together, then there should be a higher than average frequency of eating problems in people with substance abuse problems. Studies of clinical samples of alcoholics have confirmed this prediction (Lacey & Moureli, 1986; Taylor et al., 1993). In the largest study in Japan, Higuchi et al. (1993) found that 11 percent of women and 0.2 percent of men (both with alcoholism) also had an eating disorder. Bulimia nervosa was the most common problem. Additionally, the rate of eating disorders in women under 30 years of age was 72 percent. This is roughly 24 times the rate in the general population in Japan.

The only study I am aware of that studied female alcoholics from the community in addition to clinical samples was conducted by Sinha, O'Malley, Robinson, Wilson, and Rodin (1994). The subjects were 149 women, ages 18-30, with lifetime diagnoses of either alcoholism, anxiety disorders, alcoholism and anxiety disorders, or neither (controls). They were recruited from the community or outpatient clinics. Disturbed eating habits and attitudes were more common in the alcoholic women when compared with women with anxiety disorders and controls. The proportion of subjects with eating pathology was highest for the group with both alcoholism and anxiety disorders. Alcoholism was more strongly associated with severe dietary restraint and abnormal attitudes toward body shape and weight than binge eating.

FAMILY STUDIES

Clinicians have long reported high rates of substance abuse in the families of eating disorder patients. Research bears them out. The rate of substance abuse in the first-degree relatives of patients with eating disorders is higher than in the general population (Kassett et al., 1989). However, Kaye et al. (1996) found an increased rate of substance abuse only in the first-degree relatives of bulimia nervosa patients who themselves had alcohol or drug dependence. This would suggest that the two problems segregate independently in families. Particularly persuasive support for a link between binge eating and substance abuse comes from the findings that family members of both bulimia nervosa and anorexia nervosa patients with binge eating have a three- to fourfold greater lifetime risk of substance use disorders than relatives of either normal controls or restricting anorexia nervosa patients (Strober, 1995).

Studies of community samples have yielded similar findings. Garfinkel et al. (1995) found the same association in their community sample. Parents of bulimia nervosa subjects reported significantly higher lifetime rates of alcohol problems (42%) than did parents of nonpsychiatric control subjects (21%). Further evidence of a familial association between eating and alcohol problems comes from a rigorous case-control study of the development of bulimia nervosa (Fairburn et al., 1997). Parental alcohol problems emerged as a specific risk factor.

I am unaware of any study of the rate of eating disorders in the first-degree relatives of subjects with alcohol problems. Such a reciprocal relationship would be predicted if there is a strong association between the two disorders.

Once again there is no evidence of a specific association between eating and substance abuse problems in familial transmission. For example, Garfinkel et al. (1995) found that parents of bulimia nervosa subjects also had higher rates of depression, suicide attempts, and antisocial behavior than parents of nonpsychiatric controls. Moreover, when in a separate analysis the family histories of the bulimia nervosa subjects were compared with those of female subjects with lifetime depression (but not eating disorder), they found no differences.

Mechanisms Linking Eating and Substance Abuse Problems

Several explanations have been proposed but all are speculative without solid empirical support. A number of studies have shown independent familial transmission. The association between eating disorders and substance abuse does not appear to derive from a single, shared etiological factor (Kaye et al., 1996; Schuckit et al., 1996). Whatever the explanation, it will have to account for the existing findings. One is that eating disorders consistently seem to precede the onset of substance abuse problems. Moreover, patients with both disorders show an earlier onset of their substance abuse (Beary et al., 1986). The presence of an eating disorder appears to accelerate the development of substance abuse. Consistent with these findings from clinical studies, Krahn et al. (1996) found that frequency of dieting in sixth grade students predicted later alcohol intake in ninth grade.

A second is that the two disorders do not alternate over time within the same person. Successfully treated bulimia nervosa patients do not show any increase in substance abuse (Taylor et al., 1993). Symptom substitution does not occur.

Although some form of genetic/biological explanation is favored, an intriguing behavioral theory is that of reciprocal reinforcement. In laboratory studies with animals, limiting the amount of food results in the animals consistently feeding themselves alcohol. Humans, too, may increase their drug and/or alcohol use when deprived of food. This may be particularly true of persons who have bulimia nervosa because these individuals tend to eat very little between binges. This self-imposed dietary restriction could have two major effects: First, it might increase the value of highly palatable, high fat, binge foods and prompt binge eating; and second, it might increase the desirability of alternative reinforcers, such as alcohol or drugs, leading to abuse. This might explain the finding that increasing severity of dieting in female adolescents was positively associated with increasing prevalence of alcohol consumption, marijuana, and cigarette smoking (Krhan, Kurth, Demitrack, & Drewnowski, 1992).

CLINICAL RECOMMENDATIONS

Women seeking treatment for eating disorders should be routinely screened for the presence of an alcohol or drug problem. Similarly, women in treatment primarily for substance abuse problems should be assessed for an eating disorder. Studies have shown that the staff of substance abuse programs are often unaware of eating disorders in patients (Striegel-Moore et al., 1992; Taylor et al., 1993). Black and Wilson (1996) have shown that the self-report version of the Eating Disorder Examination (EDE-Q) is a brief but reliable means of assessing eating disorder psychopathology in women with substance abuse problems.

Cognitive-behavioral therapy provides effective treatment for women with binge eating and bulimia nervosa with or without a lifetime history of substance abuse (Wilson & Fairburn, 1998). In the case of binge eating patients with a current substance abuse disorder, it is my view that the latter be treated first. A sustained focus on changing eating or eliminating binge eating is impossible if there is a serious drug or alcohol problem. Once the substance abuse problem is under control, attention can then be directed to the eating problem. If the alcohol or drug abuse is not severe, it may be possible to treat the two problems at the same time.

Little is known about the effect of a co-existing eating disorder on the treatment of women in substance abuse programs. Clinical experience suggests that the eating disorder does not disappear even if the patient overcomes her substance abuse disorder. Eating disorders tend to be chronic problems. Low self-esteem is a marked characteristics of an eating disorder, and some clinicians have suggested that this increases the risk for relapse. A strong case can be made for targeting the eating disorder per se as soon as clinically feasible.

REFERENCES

American Psychiatric Association. (1994). *Diagnostic and statistical manual of mental disorders*. (4th ed.). Washington, DC: American Psychiatric Association.

Bemis, K. M. (1985). Abstinence and nonabstinence models for the treatment of bulimia. *International Journal of Eating Disorders, 4*, 407-437.

Black, C., & Wilson, G. T. (1996). Clinical interview versus self-report questionnaire in the assessment of eating disorders. *International Journal of Eating Disorders, 20*, 43-50.

Braun, D. L., Sunday, S. R., & Halmi, K. A. (1994). Psychiatric comorbidity in patients with eating disorders. *Psychological Medicine, 24*, 859-867.

Bushnell, J. A., Wells, J. E., McKenzie, J. M., Hornblow, A. R., Oakley-Browne, M. A., & Joyce, P. R. (1994). Bulimia comorbidity in the general population and in the clinic. *Psychological Medicine, 24*, 605-611.

Fairburn, C. G. (1997). Eating disorders. In D. M. Clark & C. G. Fairburn (Eds.), *The science and practice of cognitive behaviour therapy.* (pp. 209-242). Oxford: Oxford University Press.

Fairburn, C. G., Welch, S. L., Doll, H. A., Davies, B. A., & O'Connor, M. E. (1997). Risk factors for bulimia nervosa. *Archives of General Psychiatry, 54,* 509-517.

Fichter, M. M., Quadflieg, N., & Rief, W. (1994). Course of multi-impulsive bulimia, *Psychological Medicine, 24,* 591-604.

Garfinkel, P. E., Lin, E., Goering, P., Spegg, C., Goldbloom, D. S., Kennedy, S., Kaplan, A. S., & Woodside, D. B. (1995). Bulimia nervosa in a Canadian community sample: Prevalence and comparison of subgroups. *American Journal of Psychiatry, 152,* 1052-1058.

Grilo, C. M., Becker, D. F., Levy, K. N., Walker, M. L., Edell, W. S., & McGlashan, T. H. (1995). Eating disorders with and without substance use disorders: A comparative study of inpatients. *Comprehensive Psychiatry, 36,* 312-317.

Helzer, J. E., & Pryzbeck, T. R. (1988). The co-occurrence of alcoholism with other psychiatric disorders in the general population and its impact on treatment. *Journal of Studies on Alcohol, 49,* 219-224.

Higuchi, S., Suzuki, K., Yamada, K., Parrish, K., & Kono, H. (1993). Alcoholics and eating disorders: Prevalence and clinical course. *British Journal of Psychiatry, 162,* 403-406.

Holderness, C. C., Brooks-Gunn, J., & Warren, M. P. (1994). Co-morbidity of eating disorders and substance abuse review of the literature. *International Journal of Eating Disorders, 16,* 1-34.

Johnson, C. L., & Sansone, R. A. (1993). Integrating the twelve-step approach with traditional psychotherapy for the treatment of eating disorders. *International Journal of Eating Disorders, 14,* 121-134.

Kassett, J., Gershon, E., Maxwell, M., Guroff, J., Kazuba, D., Smith, A., Brandt, H., & Jimerson, D. (1989). Psychiatric disorders in the first-degree relatives of probands with bulimia nervosa. *American Journal of Psychiatry, 146,* 1468-1471.

Kaye, W. H., Lilenfeld, L. R., Plotnicov, K., Merikangas, K. R., Nagy, L., Strober, M., Bulik, C. M., Moss., H., & Greeno, C. G. (1996). Bulimia nervosa and substance dependence: Association and family transmission. *Alcohol: Clinical and Experimental Research, 20,* 878-881.

Krahn, D., Kurth, C., Demitrack, M., & Drewnowski, A. (1992). The relationship of dieting severity and bulimic behaviors to alcohol and other drug use in young women. *Journal of Substance Abuse, 4,* 341-353.

Krahn, D., Piper, D., King, M., Olson, L., Kurth, C., & Moberg, D. P. (1996). Dieting in sixth grade predicts alcohol use in ninth grade. *Journal of Substance Abuse, 8,* 293-301.

Kushner, M., Sher, K. J., & Beitman, B. (1990). The relationship between alcohol problems and the anxiety disorders. *American Journal of Psychiatry, 147,* 685-695.

Lacey, J. (1993). Self-damaging and addictive behaviour in bulimia nervosa: A catchment area study. *British Journal of Psychiatry, 163,* 190-194.

Lacey, J. H., & Moureli, E. (1986). Bulimia alcoholics: Some features of a clinical sub-group. *British Journal of Addiction, 81,* 389-393.

Laessle, R. G., Wittchen, H. U., Fichter, M. M., & Pirke, K. M. (1989). The significance of subgroups of bulimia and anorexia nervosa: Lifetime frequence of psychiatric disorders. *International Journal of Eating Disorders, 8,* 569-574.

Lilenfeld, L. R., Kaye, W. H., Greeno, C. G., Merikangas, K. R., Plotnicov, K., Pollice, C., Rao, R., Strober, M., Bulik, C. M., & Nagy, L. (1997). Psychiatric disorders in women and bulimia nervosa and their first-degree relatives: Effects of comorbid substance dependence. *International Journal of Eating Disorders, 22,* 253-264.

Marlatt, G. A., & Gordon, J. (1985). *Relapse prevention.* New York: Guilford Press.

Mitchell, J. E., & Mussell, M. P. (1995). Comorbidity and binge eating disorder. *Addictive Behaviors, 20,* 725-732.

Schuckit, M. A., Tipp, J. E., Anthenelli, R. M., Bucholz, K. K., Hesselbrock, V. M., & Nurnberger, J. I. (1996). Anorexia nervosa and bulimia nervosa in alcohol-dependent men and women and their relatives. *American Journal of Psychiatry, 153,* 74-82.

Sinha, R., Robinson, J., Merikangas, K., Wilson, G. T., Rodin, J., & O'Malley, S. (1996). Eating pathology among women with alcoholism and/or anxiety disorders. *Alcoholism: Clinical & Experimental Research, 20,* 1184-1191.

Strasser, T. J., Pike, K. M., & Walsh, B. T. (1992). The impact of prior substance abuse on treatment outcome for bulimia nervosa. *Addictive Behaviour, 17,* 387-395.

Striegel-Moore, R. H., & Huydic, E. S. (1993). Problem drinking and symptoms of disordered eating in female high school students. *International Journal of Eating Disorders, 14,* 417-426.

Strober, M. (1995). Family-genetic perspectives on anorexia nervosa and bulimia nervosa. In C. G. Fairburn & K. Brownell (Eds.), *Comprehensive textbook of eating disorders and obesity* (pp. 212-218). New York: Guilford Press.

Taylor, A. V., Peveler, R. C., Hibbert, G. A., & Fairburn, C. G. (1993). Eating disorders among women receiving treatment for an alcohol problem. *International Journal of Eating Disorders, 14,* 147-151.

Turner, M., Foggo, M., Bennie, J., Carroll, S., Dick, H., & Goodwin, G. M. (1991). Psychological, hormonal and biochemical changes following carbohydrate bingeing: A placebo controlled study in bulimia nervosa and matched controls. *Psychological Medicine, 21,* 123-133.

Walsh, B. T., Kissileff, H. R., Cassidy, S. M., & Dantzic, S. (1989). Eating behavior of women with bulimia. *Archives of General Psychiatry, 46,* 54-58.

Wardle, J. (1987). Compulsive eating and dietary restraint. *British Journal of Clinical Psychology, 26,* 47-55.

Welch, S. L., & Fairburn, C. G. (1996). Impulsivity or comorbidity in bulimia nervosa: A controlled study of deliberate self-harm and alcohol and drug misuses in a community sample. *British Journal of Psychiatry, 169,* 451-458.

Welch, S. L., & Fairburn, G. T. (1998). Smoking and bulimia nervosa. *International Journal of Eating Disorders, 23,* 433-437.

Wilson, G. T. (1993). Binge eating and addictive disorders. In C. G. Fairburn & G. T. Wilson (Eds.), *Binge eating: Nature, assessment and treatment* (97-120). New York: Guilford Press.

Wilson, G. T. (1996). Acceptance and change in the treatment of eating disorders and obesity. *Behavior Therapy, 27*, 417-439.

Wilson, G. T., & Fairburn, C. G. (1998). Treatment of eating disorders. In P. E. Nathan & J. M. Gorman (Eds.), *Psychotherapies and drugs that work: A review of the outcome studies*. New York: University Press.

Wurtman, J. (1988). Carbohydrate craving, mood changes, and obesity. *Journal of Clinical Psychiatry, 49*, 37-39.

Yanovski, S. Z., Leet, M., Yanovski, J. A., Gold, P. W., Kissileff, H. R., & Walsh, B. T. (1992). Food intake and selection of obese women with binge eating disorder. *American Journal of Clinical Nutrition, 56*, 975-980.

Yanovski, S. Z., Nelson, J. E., Dubbert, B. K., & Spitzer, R. L. (1993). Association of binge eating disorder and psychiatric comorbidity in obese subjects. *American Journal of Psychiatry, 150*, 1472-1479.

Etiology and Treatment of Obesity in Adults and Children: Implications for the Addiction Model

Risa J. Stein, PhD
Kristin Koetting O'Byrne, BA
Richard R. Suminski, PhD, MPH
C. Keith Haddock, PhD

SUMMARY. The toll obesity takes on the health of the American population is enormous. For obese children and adults the costs include impaired health and psychosocial functioning as well as staggering health care costs. It is no wonder that a plethora of treatment options have emerged in recent years. Despite the growth of the weight loss industry, no obesity treatment can claim long term efficacy for most individuals. The addictions model of obesity may offer an explanation for the disappointing outcomes of most current approaches to weight loss. According to this model, obesity is the result of a dependence on certain food substances, which obese individuals are powerless to control. Effective management of obesity, according to the addictions model, therefore includes an admission that one is powerless over food and complete absti-

Risa J. Stein is affiliated with Rockhurst University. Kristin Koetting O'Byrne is affiliated with the University of Missouri-Kansas City. Richard R. Suminski is affiliated with the University of Houston. C. Keith Haddock is Assistant Professor, Department of Psychology, University of Missouri-Kansas City and Co-Director of Behavioral Cardiology Research, Mid America Heart Institute, St. Luke's Hospital, Kansas City, MO.

Address correspondence to: Risa J. Stein, PhD, Department of Psychology, Rockhurst University, 1100 Rockhurst Road, Kansas City, MO 64110 (E-mail: R_Stein@vax1.rockhurst.edu).

[Haworth co-indexing entry note]: "Etiology and Treatment of Obesity in Adults and Children: Implications for the Addiction Model." Stein, Risa J. et al. Co-published simultaneously in *Drugs & Society* (The Haworth Press, Inc.) Vol. 15, No. 1/2, 1999, pp. 103-121; and: *Food as a Drug* (ed: Walker S. Carlos Poston II, and C. Keith Haddock) The Haworth Press, Inc., 2000, pp. 103-121. Single or multiple copies of this article are available for a fee from The Haworth Document Delivery Service [1-800-342-9678, 9:00 a.m. - 5:00 p.m. (EST). E-mail address: getinfo@haworthpressinc.com].

© 2000 by The Haworth Press, Inc. All rights reserved.

nence from offending food substances. In this paper we review the current literature on obesity etiology and the components of effective weight loss treatments and compare this literature to the major premises of the addictions model. We conclude that while the addictions model may appropriately characterize obese individuals who binge eat along some dimensions, it is inconsistent with much of what is known about the development and treatment of obesity. *[Article copies available for a fee from The Haworth Document Delivery Service: 1-800-342-9678. E-mail address: getinfo@haworthpressinc.com <Website: http://www.haworthpressinc.com>]*

KEYWORDS. Obesity, weight loss, addictions, food, dieting

Obesity among both children and adults is increasing at an alarming rate in the industrialized world. According to NHANES data, the prevalence of obesity, as defined as excess body weight (BMI > 30 kg/m^2) and/or adipose tissue (percent body fat > 25% for males or 33% for females; Baumgartner, Heymsfield, & Roche, 1995), among U.S. adults has increased 16.7% between 1960 and 1994 (Flegal, Carroll, Kuczmarski, & Johnson, 1998). The latest NHANES estimate indicates that 22.3% of U.S. adults are obese (Kuczmarski, Carroll, Flegal, & Troiano, 1997). Likewise, the prevalence of childhood obesity is at an all-time high (Epstein, 1996; Glenny, O'Meara, Melville, Sheldon, & Wilson, 1997; Haddock, Shadish, Klesges & Stein, 1994; Lifshitz, Tarim & Smith, 1993). Obesity among children has increased at least 50% since 1976 (Schonfeld-Warden & Warden, 1997). In fact, recent estimates indicate 25-27% of all children in the United States are obese as defined by a Body Mass Index (BMI) of 25 or greater (i.e., 20% above ideal body weight; Epstein, 1996). The increasing prevalence of obesity among youths is particularly striking among Native-American and Hispanic-American children (Harlan, 1993; Malina, 1993).

Given the medical consequences of obesity, the dramatic increase in the prevalence of obesity will undoubtedly place a significant burden on the public health. Obese children are at increased risk for numerous medical conditions including hyperinsulinemia, hypertension, increased triglycerides, higher levels of free fatty acids and glycerol, decreased levels of growth hormones, orthopedic problems, increased rates of intertriginous dermatitis, increased risk for respiratory tract illness, increased rates of amenorrea, dysfunctional uterine bleeding in obese girls, and atherosclerosis (Dietz, 1988; Epstein, 1996; Gerald,

Anderson, Johnson, Hoff, & Trimm, 1994; Glenny et al., 1997). An additional risk of childhood obesity is the high likelihood of becoming an obese adult. The relative risk for an obese 10-13 year old of becoming an obese adult is approximately 7 times greater than for nonobese cohorts (Epstein, 1996) and as many as 80% of obese adolescents become obese adults (Schonfeld-Warden & Warden, 1997). Moreover, adult obesity with an onset in childhood is associated with high rates of morbidity and mortality during adulthood, regardless of the level of adult adiposity (Epstein, 1996; Kennedy & Goldberg, 1995; Must, Jacques, Dallal, Bajema, & Dietz, 1992). Adults with a lifelong history of obesity are typically more obese, face more significant psychosocial problems, and are less likely to respond to treatment than individuals who were not obese as children (Mossberg, 1989).

Medical complications faced by adults who are obese include an increased risk of non-insulin dependent diabetes (Ford, Williamson, & Liu, 1997), hypertension (Dyer & Elliott, 1989), gall-bladder disease (Khare, Everhart, Maurer, & Hill, 1995), coronary heart disease (Hubert, Feinleib, McNamara, & Castelli, 1983), osteoarthritis (Cicuttini, Baker, & Spector, 1996), and various cancers (Giovannucci, Colditz, Stampfer, & Willett, 1996). The medical and social costs associated with obesity in adults are staggering, amounting to $99.2 billion in 1995 (Wolf & Colditz, 1998) and resulting in approximately 280,000 deaths per year in the United States (McGinnis & Forge, 1993).

Obese individuals are at risk not only for aversive medical consequences, but for negative psychosocial ramifications as well. Adults face discrimination as a result of obesity as well as other negative psychological consequences (Brownell & Wadden, 1992; Stunkard & Wadden, 1992). Brownell notes that "[f]or most obese persons, the psychological and social consequences of being fat are more disabling than the medical conditions" (Brownell, 1983, p. 883). Obese children have higher rates of negative peer interactions (Baum & Forehand, 1984), emotional distress (Mills & Andrianopoulos, 1993), psychiatric symptamology and depression (Mills & Andrianopoulos, 1993), lower self-esteem and body esteem (Stein, Bracken, Haddock, & Shadish, 1998), and are at increased academic risk due to discrimination from peers and school staff members (Gerald et al., 1994; Morrill, Leach, Radebaugh, & Shreeve, 1991). Gerald and colleagues (Gerald et al., 1994) state that results of social attributions of obesity may induce psychological stress and may result in higher levels of deviant behaviors among the obese.

In response to the rising tide of obesity there has been an explosion of treatment programs, diet/low fat foods, fitness centers, medications, and specially trained medical professionals all dedicated to combating excessive body weight (Poston, Foreyt, Borrell, & Haddock, 1998). Despite the voluminous attention and resources directed at the problem of obesity, its prevalence continues to climb (Foreyt & Goodrick, 1995). Ironically, the result of our increasing efforts to fight obesity has been increased rates of obesity. One explanation offered for the paradoxical relationship between the prevalence of obesity and the available resources to fight it is that most of the current methods of treating obesity involve attempts to change the patient's lifestyle and increase their self-control. Such methods, according to the addiction model, ignore the fact that obesity is due to an addictive disorder similar to alcoholism or heroin addiction (Kayloe, 1993; Yeary, 1987). The addiction model states that obese individuals are powerless to control their addiction to certain trigger foods (usually carbohydrates) and, given access to them, will eat uncontrollably.

How well does the addiction model of obesity mesh with our knowledge base regarding the etiology and treatment of obesity? In this article we will briefly review the literature on the etiology and treatment of obesity. Then we will juxtapose the scientific literature with the addiction model to assess whether conceptualizing excessive body weight as the result of an addictive disease might offer a more fruitful path to reducing the prevalence of obesity.

DOMINANT FACTORS IN THE ETIOLOGY OF OBESITY

A dominant theme in the medical literature is that obesity has no universal cause and may in fact have a heterogeneous etiology. A variety of factors may lead to an individual having a positive energy balance, that is, taking in more energy than they expend (Puhl, 1989). Generally, an individual will develop a positive energy balance from excessive caloric intake, low energy expenditure, or a combination of the two (Puhl, 1989). Thus, the literature on the etiology of obesity has focused on both physiological (e.g., genetics) and behavioral (e.g., dietary intake, physical activity) factors that result in either excessive energy intake and/or deficient energy expenditure. Below we briefly review the literature on the dominant factors in the etiology of obesity. We do not cover low-base rate causes of obesity, such as glandular abnormalities or Prader-Willi syndrome.

Genetics: The literature suggests that there are genetic influences on obesity (Stunkard, Foch, Hrubec, 1986; Stunkard, Harris, Pedersen, & McClearn, 1990). Stunkard and colleagues (1990) have reported findings of high heritability indices for BMI (66-70%; Stunkard et al., 1990) in identical twins reared apart with concordance rates significantly lower in more overweight and obese individuals than in thinner pairs of twins (36% vs. 60%, respectively; Price & Stunkard, 1989). Evidence also exists for a genetic component or components related to such important obesity-related factors as body fat distribution, basal metabolic rate, and fat cell number. While several studies clearly demonstrate a genetic contribution to obesity, it is also clear that the expression of obesity is largely dependent on behavioral and environmental factors (Foreyt & Poston, 1997). For instance, researchers have noted that obesity genetics cannot adequately explain the dramatic increases in the prevalence of obesity in industrialized countries (Foreyt & Poston, 1997; Poston & Foreyt, 1999). Moreover, Eaton and colleagues (Eaton, Konner, & Shostak, 1988a; 1988b) note that while the gene pool has not changed appreciably over the past 35,000 years, humans have dramatically changed their dietary and physical activity patterns. Thus, it is difficult to attribute the current epidemic of obesity to genetic influences.

Dietary Intake: A principal focus of much of the behavioral literature related to the etiology of obesity has been dietary intake. Three important lines of research in the dietary arena have been (1) comparing the diets of obese and lean individuals, (2) examining the role of binge eating in obesity, and (3) exploring the role of the food supply in obesity by contrasting diets cross-culturally and historically. First, do the diets of obese and lean individuals differ? While some research suggests that obese children have greater fat intake than lean children (Shah, Jeffery, Hannan, & Onstad, 1989), a majority of research finds similar daily total caloric intakes for obese and non-obese children (Epstein, 1992). For adults, however, research suggests that while both obese and lean individuals underreport their daily caloric intake, the underestimations of obese individuals approach 30–35% which is substantially greater than that of their nonobese counterparts (Heitmann

& Lissner, 1995). Thus, the overall energy intake in obese adults appears to be greater than that found for lean individuals.

While there is still debate surrounding the effect of the intake of specific macronutrients (e.g., carbohydrates) in the etiology of obesity, the scales are leaning in favor of a lack of macronutrient preference for obese individuals. For instance, although some have speculated that carbohydrate intake may play a role in the development of obesity, the prevalence of carbohydrate cravings or rate of carbohydrate consumption is not significantly different between the nonobese, obese binge eaters, and obese non-binge eaters (Goldfein, Walsh, Devlin, La-Chaussee, & Kissileff, 1992; Turner, Foggo, Bennie, Carroll, Dick, & Goodwin, 1991; Fairburn & Wilson, 1993). Moreover, even in obese individuals who binge eat, the salient feature of their binges is not cravings for specific macronutrients, but rather the amount of food eaten (Goldfein et al., 1992; Yanovski, Leet, Yanovski, Flood, Gold, Kissileff, & Walsh, 1992).

Binge eating, however, likely plays a role in the development of obesity in a subset of individuals. A history of binge eating has been found in approximately 20-30% of individuals treated in a university center while estimates of the occurrence in the general public range from approximately 5-8% (Marcus, 1995). Investigations performed in laboratory settings have found binge eaters to consume an appreciably greater amount of food than non-bingeing individuals of comparable weight (Fairburn & Wilson, 1993). This difference holds true for binges as well as during regular meals (Fairburn & Wilson, 1993). Hence, a number of studies support the role of binge eating in the development of obesity in a subset of adults (Marcus, Wing, & Hopkins, 1988; Marcus, Wing, & Lamparski, 1985; Telch, Agras, & Rossiter, 1988). In fact, binge eating is associated with even more severe adiposity (BMI = 31 – 42; Marcus, 1995).

Physical Activity. Although dietary intake has been the focus of the behavioral literature on obesity, many have argued that obesity is primarily the result of the modern sedentary lifestyle (Poston & Foreyt, 1999). The physical activity level of adults has changed dramatically across time as our country has moved from the agricultural domain into more of an industrial and now an informational realm. During the 22 years from 1965 to 1977, estimates of daily energy expenditure have dropped approximately 200 kcal per day (USDA, 1984). There is no doubt that obese adults are less physically active than nonobese adults (Brownell & Stunkard, 1980). However, Brownell and Wadden (1992) report that it is still unclear as to whether lower rates of physical activity in the obese are a factor in the etiology or a result of obesity.

A primary focus with regard to inactivity in children has been on television viewing. Dietz (1988) found that TV viewing time is one of the most powerful predictors of obesity in 6-11 year old children. Similarly, Andersen and colleagues (Andersen, Crespo, Bartlett, Cheskin, & Pratt, 1998) found that increased TV watching was associated with increased body mass index and level of body fatness. Perhaps TV viewing is related to obesity due directly to its inherently sedentary nature and indirectly to the low nutrient food typically consumed while viewing. In addition, Klesges and colleagues (Klesges, Shelton, & Klesges, 1993) found that not only is TV viewing typically incompatible with activity, but viewing may actually reduce metabolic rate. Shah and Jeffery (1991) suggest that although the history of investigations pertaining to physical activity of obese versus non-obese children is inconclusive, recent studies have begun to tip the scales in favor of the original hypothesis that obese children are less active than their lean counterparts.

Environment: The development of obesity in children may be crucially linked to their environment. In terms of family environment, children of obese parents are far more likely to become obese themselves than are children of nonobese parents (Garn & Clark, 1976; Garn, Cole, & Bailey, 1976). In fact, obesity status of parents effects the development of obesity in children from infancy through adolescence and into adulthood. Epstein and colleagues (Epstein & Cluss, 1986; Epstein, Masek, & Marshall, 1978) have suggested that parents may selectively encourage or discourage sedentary behaviors and poor nutritional habits in their children. Klesges, Coates, Moldenhauer-Klesges, Holzer, Gustavson, and Barnes (1984) have also noted that children of obese parents receive less reinforcement when they exhibit non-modeled behaviors involving physical activity.

The effects of environment on obesity also extend to one's larger culture. The culture of the United States has been described as "toxic" because of its reinforcement of unhealthy diet and activity patterns (Battle & Brownell, 1996). Like other industrialized nations, life in the United States is characterized by almost unlimited access to highly palatable and calorically dense foods (Hill & Peters, 1998). The siren call of many popular eating establishments includes phrases such as "all you can eat," "super size," and "buffet." Concurrently, most U.S. citizens experience low levels of energy expenditure during the day due to labor saving devices such as garage door openers, remote controls, elevators, and moving sidewalks. Increasingly in our information-oriented economy, individuals earn their living in sedentary occupations. Such an environment is in contradiction to the one that shaped human evolution (Poston & Foreyt, 1999).

An additional example of the effect of our toxic environment on body weight involves cultural differences in the prevalence of obesity. For instance, among Japanese men, the odds of being obese increase substantially in proportion to the proximity to the continental United States (Curb & Marcus, 1991). As the dietary fat intake of Japanese children has approached that of a typical American over the past 30 years, the prevalence of obesity has more than doubled (Murata & Hibi, 1992). Finally, rural Mexican Pima Indians who lead traditional lifestyles weigh significantly less and eat fewer calories from fat than Arizona Pima Indians who have adopted an "Americanized" diet (Ravussin, Valencia, Esparza, Bennett, & Schulz, 1994). Thus, as non-westernized people adopt American style of activity and eating, they similarly assume higher rates of weight gain and obesity. In fact, the contribution of environmental factors to body weight is so strong that Poston and Foreyt (1999) have referred to obesity as "an environmental issue" rather than a problem explained by factors within an individual patient.

In summary, the literature seems to suggest that increases in overall caloric consumption combined with reduced levels of physical activity are responsible for changes in the prevalence of obesity. Furthermore, the changes in diet and activity over time are largely due to changes in culture rather than to psychopathology, genetic defect, or physiological abnormalities within individuals.

DOMINANT TREATMENT APPROACHES FOR ADULT AND CHILDHOOD OBESITY

The variety of treatments available for obesity is staggering. Each year, a new crop of weight loss books and "miracle" treatments are marketed to an eager public willing to spend approximately $30 billion to become lean (National Task Force on the Prevention and Treatment of Obesity, 1996). Despite the plethora of treatment alternatives available to combat obesity, only two types have an adequate research base–university based behavioral programs and pharmacological interventions. Thus, we describe outcomes from clinical trials of behavioral and pharmacological interventions below as well as discuss the extant literature on addiction-model based treatment approaches.

Behavioral Programs

Behavioral treatments aim to modify eating habits and increase activity levels. A hallmark of such programs is the involvement of self-monitoring. Self-monitoring is used initially to assess deficits and strengths and subsequently to establish progress made toward goals. Most comprehensive behavioral treatments include such components as nutritional counseling, reactivation, problem-solving, focus on interpersonal relationships, cognitive restructuring, stimulus control, and relapse prevention (Wilson, 1995). Bray (1989) suggests these treatment components are based upon the following underlying assumptions: (1) an individual's eating habits as well as their exercise patterns affect body weight, (2) eating habits and exercise patterns are learned and can thus be modified using behavioral principles, and (3) long-term modification of these behaviors is dependent upon a change produced in the environment which shapes them.

The behavioral treatment of children has produced promising results. Haddock and colleagues (1994) suggest that for children and adolescents, relative to receiving no treatment at all, obesity treatments are moderately successful in reducing weight or obesity status. In their meta-analysis of childhood obesity treatments, these authors found comprehensive behavioral treatment programs which included components such as stimulus control, self-monitoring, eating management, and contingency management produced significantly better weight losses than other treatments without these components. Further, behavioral programs have demonstrated efficacy up to 10 years following treatment termination (Epstein, Valoski, & Wing, 1990). These findings are all the more salient when considering that the behavioral treatment programs work against developmental patterns of natural weight and fat gain.

Encouraging results have also been demonstrated for behavioral approaches to obesity among adults. Current behavioral treatments for obesity focus on changing diet patterns, increasing energy expenditure, and promoting the use of behavioral and cognitive modification strategies. Wing (1998) notes that in clinical trials published from 1988 to 1990 (n = 5), behavioral weight loss programs produced an average of 8.5 kg of weight loss during a 21.3 week program. At follow-up, which averaged one year, subjects maintained an average of 5.6 kg weight loss. Better maintenance of weight loss for individuals in behavioral programs is associated with longer programs, larger initial weight losses, and increased therapeutic contact during the post-treatment period (Wing, 1998).

Because individuals who receive behavioral treatment for obesity regain about 40% of their initial weight loss, a current focus of behavioral researchers is discovering strategies that enhance the long-term maintenance of weight loss. A significant factor in maintaining weight loss appears to be continued therapeutic support subsequent to termination of structured behavioral treatment programs. Perri and Fuller (1995) note that maintenance programs that include continued contact with health care providers appear to facilitate improved long-term outcomes for obese individuals. It seems adherence to eating and exercise regimens is strongly associated with continued contact with health providers. As a result, many behavioral researchers have suggested a continual care model of obesity treatment similar to that offered for diabetes.

Pharmacological Interventions

Pharmacological interventions typically are not considered a standalone treatment for obesity (USDHHS, 1998). Current guidelines for use of drugs in obesity treatment suggest that they should be used as an adjunct to behavioral interventions and only for individuals with BMIs greater than 30 or greater than 27 with concomitant medical problems (Poston et al., 1998). U.S. Federal Drug Administration approved obesity management drugs act either to reduce energy intake and increase expenditure through inhibiting serotonin and norepinephrine reuptake (Sibutramine), as a noradrenergic agent in decreasing appetite (Phentermine, Mazindol, Diethylpropion), or as a lipase inhibitor (Orlistat). Sibutramine results in weight losses of approximately 4.7 to 7.6 kg in patients engaged in clinical trials of 12 to 52 weeks (Guerciolini, 1997; Drent & van der Veen, 1993; Drent, Larsson, William-Olsson et al., 1995), while the noradrenergic drugs, usually tested in combination with dietary programs, produce mean net weight losses of approximately 2.76 ± 3.78 to 5.05 ± 2.01 kg (Ravussin et al.,

1997). Orlistat has been shown to produce moderately greater weight losses than placebo after one-year of treatment (8.76 ± 0.37 versus 5.81 ± 0.67 kg; Davidson et al., 1999). Unfortunately, for all pharmacotherapeutic agents, weight losses are promptly regained following withdrawal of the medication.

There are several shortcomings associated with the use of pharmacological agents in the treatment of obesity. First, although the majority of side-effects associated with obesity drugs are minor and seem to subside with continued use, there is the potential for serious side-effects as was noted with the use of the fenfluramine-phentermine combination (Poston et al., 1999). Issues related to potentially life-threatening repercussions of using obesity drugs has prompted the National Task Force on the Prevention of Obesity (Goldstein, Rampey, Enas, Potvin, Fludzinski, & Levine, 1994) to abstain from recommending routine pharmacotherapy for obesity treatment. Poor adherence and attrition rates constitute a second limitation of pharmacotherapy for obesity. Attrition rates as high as 85% for obesity drug therapy have been reported in clinical trials (Bray, Ryan, Gordon, Heidingsfelder, Cerise, & Wilson, 1996) and are likely to be equally high in nonclinical settings, as well. One commonly cited reason for such high attrition is the aforementioned side-effects (i.e., dry mouth, drowsiness, constipation, diarrhea) of drug treatment. The final limitation involves the difference between what most patients see as their ideal weight loss and actual weight loss on obesity medication. Poston and colleagues (Poston et al., 1999) reported that in most published studies patients only lose about 10% of their initial body weight and then by 6 months begin to plateau, and typically regain a majority of their lost weight within 6-12 months post-termination.

While there may be a place for all of the above approaches to obesity, a fourth model focusing on the traditional addiction model may provide additional direction for obesity researchers. We will now turn our attention toward an investigation of the plausibility of an addiction model in providing an explanation of adult and childhood obesity.

Obesity Treatments Based on the Addiction Model

Kay Sheppard (1989; 1993) offers a prime example of addiction model treatments for obesity. Ms. Sheppard characterizes food addiction as chronic and compulsive binge eating despite negative consequences. Food addictions, it is postulated, are formed early in childhood when refined carbohydrates are offered to children triggering the addictive process. For children predisposed to food addictions, such ingredients as sugar and food starch found frequently in many types of baby food set the stage for the development of addictive behaviors. The disease, Ms. Sheppard states, is evidenced by children seeking out enabling adults willing to provide them with their food substances of choice. The addiction theory suggests that as the child develops into adulthood, she increasingly becomes dependent on refined carbohydrates. Often, according to this model, the individuals become dependent on food items containing flour or wheat as well. The theory behind this approach suggests that individuals are powerless over certain foods as a result of the disease process. Hence, in order to control binge eating and obesity, it is first necessary to withdraw completely from the offending foods. For instance, treatment based on the food addiction model advocates abstinence from all refined carbohydrates.

One of the most popular treatment programs that is based on the addiction model is Overeaters Anonymous (OA). Although several reports have described characteristics of OA groups and their members (e.g., Maton, 1988; Weiner, 1998), systematic research regarding therapeutic benefits from OA in terms of weight loss or physiological parameters (e.g., blood pressure, lipids) are lacking. Thus, it is simply unknown whether OA or any other addiction model-based obesity treatment is efficacious. Given the large number of individuals who turn to OA for treatment of obesity, this is an alarming state of affairs. Hopefully, research on the potential therapeutic benefits of OA will occur in the future.

Although there are no data regarding the effects of therapeutic approaches based on the addiction model of obesity, studies of approaches termed "nondieting" treatments may provide some insight into the effects of programs such as OA. Nondieting approaches to obesity are typically targeted to individuals who binge eat and who suffer from greater levels of eating-related and general psychopathology than other obese patients (Goodrick, Poston, Kimball, Reeves, & Foreyt, 1998). Thus, nondieting treatments are tailored for individuals whose eating is "out-of-control" and who appear "dependent" on food to regulate their mood–individuals targeted by addiction models approaches.

Nondieting approaches to obesity focus on helping obese patients to resolve problems related to eating and body weight rather than on weight loss per se. Often gradual changes in eating and exercise patterns are recommended in a manner that is designed to be perceived as enjoyable and nonrestrictive (Goodrick et al., 1998). Unfortunately, controlled clinical trails of the nondieting approach have found it to be an unsuccessful method to achieve weight management. Individuals who complete a nondieting treatment program do not experience significant weight loss or improvements in their body dissatisfaction and do not reduce the frequency of their binge eating more than individuals who attend typical behavioral programs (e.g., Goodrick et al., 1998; Polivy & Herman, 1992). One study (Polivy & Herman, 1992) has found improvements in patients' ratings of self-esteem, eating pathology, and restraint following nondieting treatment. However, because this study was uncontrolled, it is not clear that these benefits were specific to the nondieting approach.

CONCLUSIONS

We believe that the following can be concluded regarding the addiction model of obesity:

1. The addiction model of obesity stresses dietary intake as the principal cause of obesity. In contrast, the literature on the etiology of obesity has increasingly focused on physical activity and environmental parameters as keys in the development of excess weight.
2. Although a minority of obese individuals report binge eating and feeling "out of control" during binges, most obese individuals do not report regular binge eating. Thus, at best, the addiction model only applies to a subset of obese individuals.
3. Several other key premises of the addiction model (i.e., focus on carbohydrate rich foods, requirement of abstinence from certain food substances) have received no empirical support.
4. Treatments based on the addiction model (e.g., OA) have not been empirically evaluated. Furthermore, treatment models loosely similar to the addiction model (e.g., nondieting approaches) have been evaluated and have not been found effective in treating obesity. In contrast, obesity treatment programs with the best outcomes (i.e., behavioral programs) are based on theoretical models incompatible with the addiction model (i.e., learning theory).

Thus, while it is an important exercise to seek out, investigate, apply, and evaluate potential theoretical explanations of obesity, the addiction model does not appear to provide an adequate answer to the perplexing problem of obesity.

REFERENCES

Andersen, R. E., Crespo, C. J., Bartlett, S. J., Cheskin, L. J., & Pratt, M. (1998). Relationship of physical activity and television watching with body weight and level of fatness among children: Results from the third National Health and Nutrition Examination Survey. *Journal of the American Medical Association, 279(12)*, 938-942.

Battle, E. K. & Brownell, K. D. (1996). Confronting a rising tide of eating disorders and obesity: Treatment vs. prevention and policy. *Addictive Behaviors, 21(6)*, 755-765.

Baum, C. G., & Forehand, R. (1984). Social factors associated with adolescent obesity. *Journal of Pediatric Psychology, 9(3)*, 293-302.

Baumgartner, R. N., Heymsfield, S. B., & Roche, A. F. (1995). Human body composition and the epidemiology of chronic disease. *Obesity Research, 3*, 73-95.

Bray, G. A. (1989). Classification and Evaluation of the Obesities. *Medical Clinics of North America, 73(1)*, 161-184.

Bray, G. A., Ryan, D. H., Gordon, D., Heidingsfelder, S., Cerise, F., & Wilson, K. (1996). A double-blind randomized placebo-controlled trial of sibutramine. *Obesity Research, 4*, 263-271.

Brownell, K. D. (1983). New developments in the treatments of obese children and adolescents. *Psychiatric Annals, 13(11)*, 878-883.

Brownell, K. D., & Stunkard, A. J. (1980). Physical activity in the development and control of obesity. In A. J. Stunkard (Ed.), *Obesity* (pp. 300-324). Philadelphia, PA: W. B. Sanders.

Brownell, K. D., & Wadden, T. A. (1992). Etiology and treatment of obesity: Understanding a serious, prevalent, and refractory disorder. *Journal of Consulting and Clinical Psychology, 60(4)*, 505-517.

Cicuttini, F. M., Baker, J. R., & Spector, T. D. (1996). The association of obesity with osteoarthritis of the hand and knee in women: A twin study. *Journal of Rheumatology, 23*, 1221-1226.

Curb, J. D., & Marcus, E. B. (1991). Body fat and obesity in Japanese Americans. *American Journal of Clinical Nutrition, 53*, 1552S-1555S.

Davidson, M. H., Hauptman, J., DiGirolamo, M., Foreyt, J. P., Halsted, C. H., Heber, D., Heimburger, D. C., Lucas, C. P., Robbins, D. C., Chung, J., & Heymsfield, S. B. (1999). Weight control and risk factor reduction in obese subjects treated for 2 years with Orlistat: A randomized controlled trial. *Journal of the American Medical Association, 281*, 235-242.

Dietz, W. H. (1988). Child and adolescent obesity. In R. T. Frankle and M. Yang (Eds.), *Obesity and Weight Control*. Rockville, MD: Aspen Publishers, Inc.

Drent, M. L. & van der Veen, E. A. (1993). *International Journal of Obesity and Related Metabolic Disorders, 17*, 241-244.

Drent, M. L., Larsson, I., William-Olsson, T., Quaade, F., Czubaydo, F., von Berg-mann, K., Strobel, W., Sjostrom, L., & van der Veen, E. A. (1995). Orlistat (RO 18-0647), a lipase inhibitor, in the treatment of human obesity: A multiple dose study. *International Journal of Obesity and Related Metabolic Disorders, 19,* 221-226.

Dyer, A. R., & Elliott, P. (1989). The INTERSALT study: Relations of body mass index to blood pressure. *Journal of Human Hypertension,* 3, 299-308.

Eaton, S. B., Konner, M., & Shostak, M. (1988a). Stone agers in the fast land: Chronic degenerative diseases in evolutionary perspective. *American Journal of Medicine, 84,* 739-749.

Eaton, S. B., Konner, M., & Shostak, M. (1988b). *The paleolithic prescription.* New York: Harper & Row Publishers.

Epstein, L. H. (1992). Exercise and obesity in children. *Journal of Applied Sport Psychology, 4(2),* 120-133.

Epstein, L. H. (1996). Family-based behavioural intervention for obese children. *International Journal of Obesity, 20(Suppl. 1),* S14-S21.

Epstein, L. H., & Cluss, P. A. (1986). Behavioral genetics of childhood obesity. *Behavior Therapy, 17,* 324-334.

Epstein, L. H., Masek, B. J., & Marshall, W. R. (1978). A nutritionally based school program for control of eating in obese children. *Behavior Therapy, 9,* 766-788.

Epstein, L. H., Valoski, A., & Wing, R. R. (1990). Ten-year follow-up of behavioral, family-based treatment for obese children. *Journal of the American Medical Association, 264,* 2519-2523.

Fairburn, C. G., & Wilson, G. T. (1993). *Binge eating: Nature, assessment, and treatment.* New York: Guilford Press.

Flegal, K. M., Carroll, M. D., Kuczmarski, R. J., & Johnson, C. L. (1998). Over-weight and obesity in the United States: Prevalence and trends, 1960-1994. *International Journal of Obesity, 22,* 39-47.

Ford, E. S., Williamson, D. F., & Liu, S. (1997). Weight change and diabetes inci-dence: Findings from a national cohort of US adults. *American Journal of Epide-miology,* 146, 214-222.

Foreyt, J. P., & Goodrick, G. K. (1995). Behavioral interventions in the management of obesity. *Clinical Diabetes,* 11-15.

Foreyt, J. P., & Poston, W. S. C. (1997). Diet, genetics, and obesity. *Food Technology, 51,* 7073.

Garn, S. M., Cole, P. E., & Bailey, S. M. (1976). Effect of parental fatness levels on the fatness of biological and adoptive children. *Ecology of Food and Nutrition, 6,* 1-3.

Garn, S. M., & Clark, D. C. (1976). Trends in fatness and the origins of obesity. *Pediatrics, 57,* 433-456.

Gerald, L. B., Anderson, A., Johnson, G. D., Hoff, C., & Trimm, R. F. (1994). Social class, social support and obesity risk in children. *Child: Care, health and develop-ment, 20,* 145-163.

Giovannucci, E., Colditz, G. A., Stampfer, M. J., & Willett, W. C. (1996). Physical activity, obesity, and risk of colorectal adenema in women (United States). *Cancer Causes Control, 7,* 253-263.

Glenny, A. M., O'Meara, S., Melville, A., Sheldon, T. A., & Wilson, C. (1997). The treatment and prevention of obesity: A systematic review of the literature. *International Journal of Obesity, 21*, 715-737.

Goldfein, J., Walsh, B. T., Devlin, M. J., LaChaussee, J., & Kissileff, H. (1992). *Eating behavior in binge eating disorder.* Paper presented at the fifth International Conference on Eating Disorders, New York.

Goldstein, D. J., Rampey, A. H. J., Enas, G. G., Potvin, J. H., Fludzinski, L. A., & Levine, L. R. (1994). Fluoxetine: A randomized clinical trial in the treatment of obesity. *International Journal of Obesity, 18*, 129-135.

Goodrick, G. K., Poston, W. S. C., Kimball, K. T., Reeves, R. S., & Foreyt, J. P. (1998). Nondieting versus dieting treatment for overweight binge-eating women. *Journal of Consulting and Clinical Psychology, 66*, 363-368.

Guerciolini, R. (1997). Mode of action of orlistat. *International Journal of Obesity and Related Metabolic Disorders, 21(S3)*, S12-S23.

Haddock, C. K., Shadish, W. R., Klesges, R. C., & Stein, R. J. (1994). Treatments for childhood and adolescent obesity. *Annals of Behavioral Medicine, 16(3)*, 235-244.

Harlan, W. R. (1993). Epidemiology of childhood obesity. *Annals of the New York Academy of Science, 699*, 1-5.

Heitman, B. L., & Lissner, L. (1995). Dietary underreporting by obese individuals: Is it specific or non-specific? *British Medical Journal, 311*, 986-989.

Hill, J. O. & Peters, J. C. (1998). Environmental contributions to the obesity epidemic. *Science, 280*, 1371-1374.

Hubert, H. B., Feinleib, M., McNamara, P. M. & Castelli, W. P., (1983). Obesity as an independent risk factor for cardiovascular disease: A 26-year follow-up of participants in the Framingham Heart Study. *Circulation, 67(5)*, 968-977.

Kayloe, J. C. (1993). Food addiction. *Psychotherapy, 30*, 269-275.

Kennedy, E., & Goldberg, J. (1995). What are American children eating? Implications for Public Policy. *Nutrition Reviews, 53(5)*, 111-126.

Khare, M., Everhart, J. E., Maurer, K. R., & Hill, M. C. (1995). Association of ethnicity and body mass index (BMI) with gallstone disease in the United States. *American Journal of Epidemiology, 141*, S69.

Klesges, R. C., Coates, T. J., Moldenhauer-Klesges, L. M., Holzer, B., Gustavson, J., & Barnes, J. (1984). The fats: An observational system for assessing physical activity in children and associated parent behavior. *Behavioral Assessment, 6*, 333-345.

Klesges, R. C., Shelton, M. L. & Klesges, L. M. (1993). Effects of television on metabolic rate: Potential implications for childhood obesity. *Pediatrics, 91*, 281-286.

Kuczmarski, R. J., Carroll, M. D., Flegal, K. M., Troiano, R. P. (1997). Varying body mass index cutoff points to describe overweight prevalence among U.S. adults: NHANES III (1988 to 1994). *Obesity Research, 5(6)*, 542-548.

Lifshitz, F., Tarim, O., & Smith, M. M. (1993). Nutrition in adolescence. *Adolescent Endocrinology, 22(3)*, 673-683.

Malina, R. M. (1993). Ethnic variation in the prevalence of obesity in North American children and growth. *Critical Reviews in Food, Science, and Nutrition, 33*, 389-396.

Marcus, M. D. (1995). Binge eating and obesity. In K. D. Brownell & C. G. Fairburn (Eds.), *Eating disorders and obesity: A comprehensive handbook*. New York: Guilford Press.

Marcus, M. D., Wing, R. R., & Hopkins, J. (1988). Obese binge eaters: Affect, cognitions, and response to behavioral weight control. *Journal of Consulting and Clinical Psychology, 56*, 433-439.

Marcus, M. D., Wing, R. R., & Lamparski, D. (1985). Binge eating and dietary restraining in obese patients. *Addictive Behaviors, 10*, 163-168.

Maton, K. I. (1989). Towards a ecological understanding of mutual-help groups: The social ecology of "fit." *American Journal of Community Psychology, 17*, 729-753.

McGinnis, J. M., & Forge, W. H. (1993). Actual causes of death in the United States. *Journal of the American Medical Association, 270*, 2207-2212.

Mills, J. K., & Andrianopoulos, G. D. (1993). The relationship between childhood onset obesity and psychopathology in adulthood. *Journal of Psychology, 127*, 547-551.

Morrill, C. M., Leach, J. N., Radebaugh, M. R., & Shreeve, W. C. (1991). Adolescent Obesity: Rethinking Traditional Approaches. *The School Counselor, 38*, 347-351.

Mossberg, H. O. (1989). 40-year follow-up of overweight children. *Lancet, 2*, 491-493.

Murata, M. & Hibi, I. (1992). Nutrition and the secular trend of growth. *Hormone Research, 38(S1)*, 89-96.

Must, A., Jacques, P. F., Dallal, G. E., Bajema, C. J., & Dietz, W. H. (1992). Long-term morbidity and mortality of overweight adolescents: A follow-up of the Harvard Growth Study of 1922-1935. *New England Journal of Medicine, 237*, 1350-1355.

National Task Force on the Prevention and Treatment of Obesity. (1996). Long-term pharmacotherapy in the management of obesity. *Journal of the American Medical Association, 276*, 1907-1915.

Perri, M. G. & Fuller, P. R. (1995). Success and failure in the treatment of obesity: Where do we go from here? *Medicine, Exercise, Nutrition and Health, 5(4)*, 255-272.

Polivy, J., & Herman, C. P. (1992). Undieting: A program to help people stop dieting. *International Journal of Eating Disorders, 11*, 261-268.

Poston, W. S. C. & Foreyt, J. P. (In press). Obesity is an environmental issue, *Atherosclerosis*.

Poston, W. S. C., Foreyt, J. P., Borrell, L. & Haddock, C. K. (1998). Challenges in obesity management. *Southern Medical Journal, 91*, 710-720.

Puhl, J. L. (1989). Energy expenditure among children: Implications for childhood obesity I: Resting and dietary energy expenditure. *Pediatric Exercise Science, 1*, 212-229.

Price, R. A., & Stunkard, A. J. (1989). Commingling analysis of obesity in twins. *Human Heredity, 39(3)*, 121-135.

Ravussin, E., Pratley, R. E., Maffej, M., Wang, H., Friedman, J. M., Bennett, P. H., & Bogardus, C. (1997). Relatively low plasma leptin concentrations precede weight gain in Pima Indians. *National Medicine, 3*, 238-240.

Ravussin, E., Valencia, M. E., Esparza, J., Bennett, P. H., & Schulz, L. O. (1994). Effects of a traditional lifestyle on obesity in Pima Indians. *Diabetes Care, 17*, 1067-1074.

Schonfeld-Warden, N., & Warden, C. H. (1997). Pediatric obesity: An overview of etiology and treatment. *Pediatric Clinics of North America, 44*, 339-361.

Shah, M. & Jeffrey, R. W. (1991). Is obesity due to overeating and inactivity, or to a defective metabolic rate? A review. *Annals of Behavioral Medicine, 13(2)*, 73-79.

Shah, M., Jeffery, R. W., Hannan, P. J., & Onstad, L. (1989). The relationship between sociodemographic and behavior variables and body mass index in a population with high-normal blood pressure: Hypertension Prevention Trial. *European Journal of Clinical Nutrition, 43*, 583-596.

Sheppard, K. (1989). *Food addiction: The body knows.* Deerfield Beach, FL: Health Communications, Inc.

Sheppard, K. (1993). *Food addiction: The body knows (rev/expanded ed.)* Deerfield Beach, FL: Health Communications, Inc.

Stein, R. J., Bracken, B. R., Haddock, C. K., & Shadish, W. R. (1998). Preliminary development of the Children's Physical Self-Concept Scale. *Journal of Developmental and Behavioral Pediatrics, 19*, 1-18.

Stunkard, A. J., Foch, T. T., Hrubec, Z. (1986). A twin study of human obesity. *Journal of the American Medical Association, 256(1)*, 51-54.

Stunkard, A. J., Harris, J. R., Pedersen, N. L., & McClearn, G. E. (1990). A separated twin study of the body mass index. *New England Journal of Medicine, 322*, 1483-1487.

Stunkard, A. J., & Wadden, T. A. (1992). Psychological aspects of severe obesity. *American Journal of Clinical Nutrition, 55 (2S)*, 524S-532S.

Telch, C. F., Agras, W. S., & Rossiter, E. M. (1988). Binge eating increases with increasing adiposity. *International Journal of Eating Disorders, 7*, 115-119.

Turner, M. St. J., Foggo, M., Bennie, J., Carroll, S., Dick, H., & Goodwin, G. M. (1991). Psychological, hormonal and biochemical changes following carbohydrate bingeing: A placebo controlled study in bulimia nervosa and matched controls. *Psychological Medicine, 21*, 123-133.

U.S. Department of Agriculture. (1984). *Nationwide food consumption survey. Nutrient intakes, individuals in 48 states, year 1977-1978.* Report No. 1-2, Consumer Nutrition Division, Human Nutrition Information Service, Hyattsville, MD.

U.S. Department of Health and Human Services (1998). *Clinical guidelines on the identification, evaluation, and treatment of overweight and obesity in adults: The evidence report.* Washington, DC: U.S. Government Printing Office.

Weiner, S. (1988). The addiction of overeating: Self-help groups as treatment models. *Journal of Clinical Psychology, 54*, 163-167.

Wilson, G. T. (1995). Eating disorders and addictive disorders. In K. D. Brownell & C. G. Fairburn (Eds.), *Eating disorders and obesity: A comprehensive handbook.* New York: Guilford Press.

Wing, R. R. (1998). Behavioral approaches to the treatment of obesity. In G. A. Bray, C. Bouchard, & W. P. T. James (Eds.) *Handbook of Obesity.* New York: Marcel Dekker, Inc.

Wolf, A. M., & Colditz, G. A. (1998). Current estimates of the economic costs of obesity in the United States. *Obesity Research, 6,* 97-106.

Yanovski, S. Z., Leet, M., Yanovski, J. A., Flood, M., Gold, P. W., Kissileff, H. R., & Walsh, B. T. (1992). Food selection and intake of obese women with binge eating disorder. *American Journal of Clinical Nutrition, 56,* 975-980.

Yeary, J. (1987). The use of Overeaters Anonymous in the treatment of eating disorders. *Journal of Psychoactive Drugs, 19,* 303-309.

Inability to Control Eating:
Addiction to Food or Normal Response
to Abnormal Environment?

G. Ken Goodrick, PhD

SUMMARY. Both the increasing prevalence of obesity in a society obsessed with trying to be thin, and the self-reported inability to control
eating in many obese patients, point to the possibility that overeating
may be prevalent despite attempts to control it. The apparent lack of
control has led some to describe overeating as an addiction. This paper
briefly reviews the problem of overeating by examining the associated
phenomenological, psychological, and physiological correlates of excessive appetite. A variety of factors may contribute to overeating, including the food environment, social influence, use of food to alleviate
negative mood states, and potentiation of appetite from restrictive dieting. Although overeating may not fit an addictive model, the lack of
self-control over eating has implications for treatment interventions and
public health policy. *[Article copies available for a fee from The Haworth Document Delivery Service: 1-800-342-9678. E-mail address: getinfo@haworthpress
inc.com <Website: http://www.haworthpressinc.com>]*

KEYWORDS. Compulsive eating, addiction, restrictive dieting, overeating, obesity

---

G. Ken Goodrick is affiliated with the Behavioral Medicine Research Center,
Baylor College of Medicine.

Address correspondence to: G. Ken Goodrick, PhD, Behavioral Medicine Research Center, Baylor College of Medicine, 6535 Fannin F700, Houston, TX 77030
(E-mail: goodrick@bcm.tmc.edu).

Preparation of this paper was supported in part by Grant DK48463 from the
National Institute of Diabetes, Digestive and Kidney Diseases.

[Haworth co-indexing entry note]: "Inability to Control Eating: Addiction to Food or Normal Response
to Abnormal Environment?" Goodrick, G. Ken. Co-published simultaneously in *Drugs & Society* (The
Haworth Press, Inc.) Vol. 15, No. 1/2, 1999, pp. 123-140; and: *Food as a Drug* (ed: Walker S. Carlos Poston
II, and C. Keith Haddock) The Haworth Press, Inc., 2000, pp. 123-140. Single or multiple copies of this
article are available for a fee from The Haworth Document Delivery Service [1-800-342-9678, 9:00 a.m. - 5:00
p.m. (EST). E-mail address: getinfo@haworthpressinc.com].

© 2000 by The Haworth Press, Inc. All rights reserved.

OVERVIEW

The prevalence of obesity in the United States is increasing rapidly (Kuczmarksi, Flegal, Campbell, & Johnson, 1994); it has been predicted, based on trends over the last few decades, that all adults will be obese by the year 2230 (Foreyt & Goodrick, 1995). While many assume that this increasing prevalence is caused by increased consumption of calories, there is evidence that the main culprit may be lack of exercise (Bennett, 1995). However, given the low level of physical activity in modern industrialized nations, the amount of calories eaten does give rise to increased weight. This may be abetted by the increase in calorie density in the food environment (Poppitt & Prentice, 1996), rather than the actual amount of food eaten. It should be remembered that in the original behavior modification studies of weight management, subjects who claimed to be overeating could not finish low-calorie density meals designed to meet their metabolic needs, indicating that they were used to a higher calorie-density regimen (Stuart, 1967).

For the health professional dealing with obesity or eating disorders, the problem is how to help the patient who reports lack of control over eating. The feeling of being out of control is distressing, because the patient feels that he or she should be able to control calorie intake; failure to do so is viewed as a lack of willpower or character. Our cultural traditions in the Western world stem from thousands of years of teachings defining a good person as one in whom the mind has control over the base instincts. As Cicero said, "Reason should direct and appetite obey." Obesity is often taken as a sign of personal failing. In preindustrial society, obesity was a sign of sloth and/or gluttony compared to all others who had to toil for a living, and who were too poor to overindulge in food. Even though about one-third of the population is overweight, and the causes of obesity are clearly not associated with personal character, the stigma against the obese remains.

One answer to this problem for some is to view obesity as the result of a disease characterized by lack of control over eating, or as an *addiction*. Although "addiction" is not clearly defined in medicine or psychiatry, the concept allows patients to view themselves as victims of physiological processes which are not their fault. The problems with this model of overeating as a disease have been thoroughly reviewed by Wilson (1991). The "symptoms" of the disease include perceived loss of eating control, cravings, preoccupation with food, and sometimes denial and secrecy. Overeating is alternated with restrictive dieting, and eating is used to regulate emotions and to cope with stress in a manner similar to the use of psychotropic drugs. However, these symptoms can be better explained as the result of normal physiological processes in the control of eating in response to the very abnormal situation of the modern human. This abnormal situation includes:

- Sedentary behavior patterns
- Abundance of high-calorie density food
- A natural facility for weight gain as an adaptive physiological response
- A strong desire to control weight
- A dependence upon restrictive dieting to control weight
- Psychophysiological responses to dieting which enhance appetite
- Periodic loss of control of eating with weight gain
- Feelings of inadequacy due to the perception that one should be able to control eating.

This describes the well-known "dieters dilemma" (Bennett & Gurin, 1982).

As Wilson (1991) points out, there is no evidence for a "biological vulnerability," or an "addictive personality," or for foods (e.g., white flour, sugar) which can precipitate an addictive, uncontrolled eating response. Further, he points out that the so-called uncontrollable eating behaviors do seem to be under control when subjected to social scrutiny; bingers will not binge if they know they are to be observed by those who know about their eating problems. This is an important point which will be considered below with respect to implications for treatment and public health interventions.

If eating dyscontrol is not an addiction, then what is it? Much of the overweight public perceives it as a problem which is not amenable to self-control. The demand for appetite suppressant medication is very high. Sales of nutritional supplements for appetite control, and for devices which claim to help in weight control continue to rise. Many of the overweight have struggled for years, only to see their weight slowly increase; it is no wonder that they perceive themselves as out of control, and needing a "magic pill." At the same time, therapists are struggling to get patients to alter their eating and exercise habits towards a new, permanent lifestyle, which most seem to abandon within a few years, based on the regain likely for the vast majority of those so treated.

The problem is in part due to the culturally-based perception that certain behaviors are controllable through "willpower" or volition. In fact they are in large part controlled by physiological processes which are not well connected to those parts of the brain associated with thought and rational action. Table 1 shows basic functions for which there is a disparity between perceived and actual degree of control.

The functions shown (eating, breathing, sleep, sex, and exercise) are necessary for species survival, and therefore they can be expected to have strong underlying physiological support for their occurrence. For each function, humans construe the associated behaviors to be, in varying degrees, under the control of both cognitive and physiological processes. Whereas most people recognize that breathing and sleeping are not to be denied, due to the primacy of physiological control, the perception is that eating can be controlled. Overweight individuals' attempts to control weight through restrictive dieting apparently involve the assumption that they can control their eating. However, eventually they come to the realization that much of their eating is out of their cognitive control. (Physiological correlates for this are described later.) Those with weight fluctuations due to periodic dieting (motivated by greater body dissatisfaction) are more likely to have

TABLE 1. Perceived vs. Actual Control of Species Survival Functions

Survival Function		Relative Degree of Control		
		Cognitive	< - - - - - >	Physiological
Eating	Perceived	X (norm.)		X (hx dieting)
	Actual		X (norm.)	X (hx dieting)
Breathing	Perceived		X	
	Actual			X
Sleep	Perceived			X
	Actual			X
Sex	Perceived	X		
	Actual			X
Exercise	Perceived	X		
	Actual	(high fitness compels exercise)		X
		(low fitness compels rest)		X

lower levels of self-efficacy for eating control (Toray & Cooley, 1997). The perceived psychological control of eating may be more epiphenomenal to eating behaviors than they are causal. The problem is that these perceptions lead to feelings of inadequacy in the case of eating, while the apparent inability to restrict breathing would not be viewed as a character flaw. Indeed, overeating after restrictive dieting is analogous to gasping for air after restricted breathing; few would regard this as a failure of "willpower."

Implicit in Table 1 is that "cognitive" control and "physiological control" are separate processes. However, they are interactive. For example, cognitive activities concerning food (thoughts, viewing of food pictures) can change physiological processes associated with increased appetite, such as pancreatic reflex discharge of insulin and glucagon (Bellisle, 1995). Physiological events, such as drop in blood sugar associated with insulin increase, precipitate cognitions of food which lead to eating (Campfield, Smith, Rosenbaum, & Hirsch, 1996). The affective perception of a food stimulus changes as a function of the internal energy status; a pleasant food becomes less pleasant after much of it is eaten (Bellisle, 1995). The classic mind-body problem thus blurs our ability to describe the nexus of causality in eating control. The situation becomes more complex with the realization that mental activities, and control of eating behavior, operate to a large extent under the influence of the physical and social environment.

Another interesting point should be made from Table 1, especially as lack of exercise may be primary in the increasing prevalence of obesity, along with eating control problems. Whether a person exercises or not is seen as under high volitional control. However, there is a physiological control component. Those who are sedentary have low physical fitness, which means that they feel less energetic, and a given amount of exercise may seem more burdensome. This can be construed as a negative physiological influence. However, those who exercise regularly feel more energetic, are more likely to exercise due to feelings of energy, and perceive exercise to be enjoyable (e.g., Riddle, 1980; Goodrick, Malek, & Foreyt, 1994). Not only that, but physically fit people report irritability and negative mood if they are prevented from exercising; to that extent exercise behavior is subject to a positive physiological influence.

PSYCHOLOGY OF ATTEMPTS TO CONTROL EATING

Virtually all patients presenting for weight management treatment have a history of restrictive dieting attempts. Thus, when dealing with these individuals, one must examine the psychological and physiological correlates of restricted eating. Studies of human starvation (Keys, Brozek, & Henschel, 1950) have shown that when men are reduced to 76% of original body weight through limited diet, they become preoccupied with thoughts of food, and become depressed and irritable. About half the subjects in this study reported that food was still a preoccupation for them long after the study was over, and that they had established eating behaviors that had the character of rituals. It is not surprising that women, who comprise the vast majority of patients in weight management programs, and who may be more sensitive to weight concerns because of cultural influences (Foreyt & Goodrick, 1982; Brownell, 1991a; 1991b), develop a strained relationship with food and dieting. Dieting may give rise to a preoccupation with food, and attempts to suppress such thoughts in order to gain eating control may actually lead to an increase in such thoughts, and failure of eating control (Ward, Bulik, & Johnston, 1996). Severe dieting, such as very low calorie diets, may cause some patients to become binge eaters (Telch & Agras, 1993).

Clinical experience and research (Sjöberg & Persson, 1979) show that when those with weight concerns attempt to control eating using restrictive diets, they often arrive at a psychophysiological state characterized by an apparent conflict between desires to lose weight and compulsion to eat. This state includes muddled thinking about original weight-loss goals, and eating discordant with intention (Ruderman, 1986). Overeating may result from a motivated shift to lower levels of self-awareness, as an escape from painful feelings of personal inadequacy (Heatherton & Baumeister, 1991). Relapses from diet regimens seem to occur upon exposure to food at mealtime, either when socializing or when alone, when happy, tense, angry, or depressed, or when bored (Grilo, Shiffman & Wing, 1989). Over-eating often seems to be an activity done in response to emotional distress, or to the perception that one has "blown" a diet by eating some forbidden food (Heatherton, Polivy, & Herman, 1990).

For the non-dieting person without weight concerns, and without restricted access to food, eating is perceived to be largely under psychological control, even though the regularity of eating may indicate that physiological processes actually dominate. For individuals with weight concerns who have a history of dieting, their experience with relapse from diet regimens may lead them to believe that eating is psychologically "out-of-control," and totally under the control of psychophysiological forces they cannot master. This is generally the scenario when patients present for weight management therapy (Goodrick & Foreyt, 1991).

Table 2 depicts the three most common conditions for overeating: negative emotions, boredom, and happy, social situations. The possible reinforcement mechanisms to explain overeating include enjoyment, which might be beneficial for each of the three conditions. Overeaters report that binge eating helps to alleviate negative emotions (Greeno & Wing, 1994; Kuehnel & Wadden, 1994). Some patients report that cooking and eating are good distractions from negative emotional states, but there is little research on this. As mentioned above, some overeating seems to take on the characteristics of an altered state of consciousness, which focuses so intensely on eating that the pain of low self-esteem is temporarily forgotten (Heather & Baumeister, 1991). Patients typically say that boredom can precipitate eating, and overeating at social events may be due to behavioral contagion influences interacting with the sensation of food.

There are two problems with situational/affective explanations of overeating. One is that there are so many potential conditions associated with overeating, that any theory explaining overeating as a function of such conditions suffers from the problem of a continuous anteced-

TABLE 2. Rationales for Overeating/Diet Relapse

Putative Reinforcement	Negative Emotions	Boredom	Positive Emotions– Social Situations
Enjoyment	C	C	C
Anti-Depressant	OD		
Distraction	C		
Escape from Self-Awareness	C		
Stimulation		C	
Behavioral Contagion			P

C = Cephalic phase effect: sensory
OD = Neurotransmitter effect: opioid, dopaminergic
P = Psychological effect

ent. In other words, for a theory to be predictively valid, it must specify a narrow set of conditions associated with observations. If overeating is associated with negative and positive emotions, as well as no affect (boredom), then the concept of affect-induced overeating, sometimes referred to as the narrower concept of negative affect-induced eating (NAIE), is not very useful. The other problem is that most research on emotional/situational overeating uses retrospective methodology, which may be subject to self-justification biases and the demand characteristics of the study (Faith, Wong, & Allison, 1998).

In summary, patients who report problems in eating control most likely have a history of restrictive dieting, which may potentiate psychological aspects of appetite. They report eating as a form of self-medication for negative affective states, and also in response to social influences with positive affective states. All this occurs in an environment of abundant food, much of which has been processed to maximize appetite. When rats are placed into such an environment, they eat more and become obese, but they are not motivated to try to control themselves to avoid stigmatization. Many humans placed into such an environment (the industrialized world) present with the complaint of obesity and report the perception that they can't control their eating; indeed, some feel they are "addicted" to food.

Before making a jump to any conclusions about the nature of overeating, an examination is in order of the physiological evidence which helps to explain the apparent disparity between desire for eating control and hyperphagia.

PHYSIOLOGICAL REWARD PATHS OF EATING

Parallels have been drawn between overeating and drug addiction, since both behavioral syndromes involve intense cravings and loss of self-control. There may be similar physiological mechanisms which mediate both food and drug reward. For example, sweet cravings are associated with opiate addiction (Willenbring, Morley, Krahn, Carlson, Levine & Shafer, 1989), and opiate withdrawal is often eased by eating of sweets (Morabia, Fabre, Chee, Zeger, Orsat, & Robert, 1989). The opiate antagonist naloxone has been shown to reduce taste preferences, and reduced calorie intake from snacks in binge eaters; preferences for sweet, high-fat foods were especially affected (Drewnowski, Krahn, Demitrack, Nairn, & Gosnell, 1992). Since binge eaters report a pattern of compulsive overeating that can be triggered by such palatable foods, and since the eating seems to alleviate some negative mood states, the parallel to drug dependence is compelling.

As discussed above, most patients presenting with the complaint of uncontrolled eating have a history of restrictive dieting. Food deprivation increases the reward value of food (Berridge, 1991), possibly by sensitizing the opioid reward system (Carr & Simon, 1984). Multiple episodes of food restriction, typical of dieting in humans, make rats supersensitive to the effects of the appetite-stimulating effect of brain opioids, through mechanisms which may overlap those associated with opioid involvement in drug addiction (DeVry, Donselaar, & Van Ree, 1989; Carr & Papadouka, 1994). Obese humans characterized by large weight fluctuations (presumably from bouts of restrictive dieting) show elevated preferences for sugar and fat mixtures compared to obese persons with stable weight (Drewnowski, Kurth, & Rahaim, 1991). From an adaptive viewpoint, it makes sense that an animal would want to eat more after a period of starvation, to make up for lost weight. However, the potentiation of eating seems to persist even after normal weight is regained (Hagan & Moss, 1991), setting the stage for obesity as a long-term outcome of restrictive dieting. Overeating after restrictive dieting may also be due to feedback signals from lean and fat tissues. Unfortunately, dieters typically regain lost fat faster than they regain lost fat-free mass (FFM), so that when fat mass is restored, there is still a hunger signal due to reduced FFM; the resultant eating also adds to the fat mass, making the post-diet individual fatter than before a diet (Dulloo, Jacquet, & Girardier, 1997).

Hoebel (1997a) has reviewed the research on neuroscience and appetite, attempting to show how physiological processes result in eating behavior. He notes that opioid peptides may have a special role in prolonging a meal, resulting in more calories being eaten; this may explain the (opioid-mediated) preference for dessert even after a big meal. An animal model of "food addiction" was developed by Hoebel (1997b) by training rats to binge with daily access to glucose solutions which they drank in increasing amounts. When they were subsequently deprived of food for one or two days, they exhibited withdrawal symptoms (teeth chattering and paw fanning). These symptoms were augmented with naloxone, or reversed by morphine. Thus periodic bingeing may lead to augmented eating, followed by opioid withdrawal during subsequent deprivation. The binge eating caused significant changes in opioid receptor binding in certain areas of the brain, notably the accumbens (Colatuoni, McCarthy, Gibbs, Searls, Alisharan, & Hoebel, 1997). Binge eating may be reduced with opiate antagonists (Mitchell, Laine, Morley, & Levine, 1986).

The dopamine (DA) reward theory posits that DA release in the nucleus accumbens (NAc) reinforces any behavior, and acetylcholine (ACh) inhibits behavior. Opioid links have been identified in this eating reward circuit which projects from the hypothalamus to the NAc. Food deprivation lowers DA levels in the NAc, and raises ACh (Pothos, Creese, & Hoebel, 1995). This led Hoebel (1997a) to speculate that during food restriction (dieting) alternative behaviors such as binge eating or drug abuse may occur to restore DA levels. The sights, sounds, and smells of food may also trigger DA release through conditioning (Schultz, Dayan, & Motague, 1997), thus potentiating eating in an environment filled with food stimuli (i.e., modern society). Treatment with DA agonists may be helpful in the treatment of obesity, by reducing the amount of food consumption needed to obtain a satisfying level of DA in the brain (Cincotta, Tozzo, & Scislowski, 1997; Cincotta & Meier, 1996).

OVEREATING AS AN ADDICTION versus A NATURAL RESPONSE TO AN UNNATURAL CULTURE

Hoebel (1997b) points out that there are three steps to becoming addicted:

1. Behavioral sensitization phase: an increase in intake of the substance.
2. Withdrawal phase: abstaining from substance use causes symptoms that are very unpleasant.
3. Craving phase: a long-lasting, strong appetite for the substance that leads to loss of control and relapse to more substance use.

According to Hoebel (1997b), the hallmark of addiction is long-term neural change that creates the loss of control. Changes in opioid reward activation as discussed above might be taken as evidence for an addictive process based on physiological changes. However, it is not clear that discovery of physiological reward pathways proves that overeating is an "addictive" disorder, caused by a "disease" that requires treatment of an individual. It does show that humans, like other mammals, are programmed for species survival to eat (and breathe and breed and sleep). Part of this programming can be adjusted to compensate for variations in food availability. The changes associated with restrictive dieting, together with the appetite-stimulating modern food environment of abundant, highly palatable foods, lead many to perceive themselves as lacking in self-control.

Nonetheless, *"self*-control" is an inappropriate label if one recognizes that eating is ultimately controlled by physiological/behavioral/environmental/social relationships. It can be argued that if the environmental and social factors are adjusted, then eating will be under apparent "self" control. For example, there are numerous examples of the increases in inappropriate eating and insufficient exercise caused by the translocation of peoples from primitive to modern cultures (Foreyt & Poston, 1997), and of the restoration of more healthful lifestyles by relocation back to more primitive conditions (O'Dea, 1991).

A simplistic model of the factors related to eating is shown in Figure 1. In this model, "appetite" is defined as the profile of psychophysiological conditions which are normally associated with eating behavior. However, the "decision to eat," while influenced by food stimuli and physiological factors, is also subject to the influence of sociocultural learning, which may potentiate the effect of social scrutiny on eating. For example, few obese binge-eating women will binge

FIGURE 1. Factors Involved in Eating Control

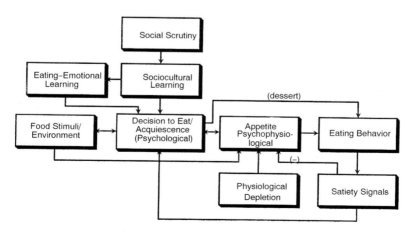

in front of non-bingeing friends. As Wilson (1991) points out, bulimics will not overeat if they are in a situation which forbids purging. Social support is important in weight management efforts, as shown by retrospective reports (Kayman, Bruvold, & Stern, 1990; Klem, Wing, McGuire, Seagle, & Hill, 1998), and by the finding that interpersonal therapy, which helps patients to develop better relationships, seems to be effective for treatment of bulimia (Fairburn, Jones, Peveler, Hope, & O'Connor, 1993).

The importance of the food environment cannot be underemphasized as one cause of overeating in modern industrialized society. In natural settings, food supply and eating are limited by the establishment of territories for most animals. Within a territory, if a squirrel eats some nuts, the supply of nuts is thereby diminished. However, for most humans in the industrialized world, the situation is quite different. Figure 2 shows the feedback associated with the eating of chips (as a high-calorie-density example). When consumers eat more chips, the increased market demand leads the food industry to increase varieties, make larger displays (currently more than one aisle at some grocery stores), and increase advertising in the media. At the same time, competitive forces from new chip makers may drive prices down. All of these changes increase the probability of chip eating among consumers.

Consumption patterns in developing countries, and in countries

FIGURE 2. Effect of Eating on Food Environment

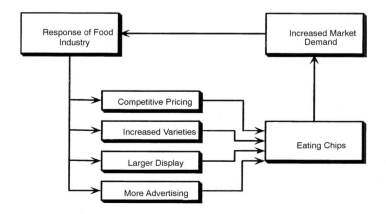

which have traditionally low-calorie-dense diets, are changing in the direction of increasing the probability of overeating and increasing the prevalence of obesity. For example, as American fried chicken, hamburger and pizza restaurants proliferate in the Far East, consumption of rice has declined 50 percent in Japan and Taiwan over the last 30 years (International Food Policy Research Institute, 1998).

These trends can be reversed. In the Minjilang Project, in an Aboriginal village on an island off northern Australia, the quality of the food supply at the community store was improved substantially, with greater emphasis on fruits and vegetables, and a reduction in sugar and meat fat. This resulted in a general reduction in serum cholesterol and weight in the community (Lee, Bailey, Yarmirr, O'Dea, & Mathews, 1994). Another study examined the effects of transporting Aboriginal Australians, who were suffering from obesity and diabetes due to a Western lifestyle, back to their native conditions (O'Dea, 1991). Here again, obesity, diabetic complications, and cardiovascular risk factors declined without requiring much "self-control." This brings to mind studies of those who first used "addictive" drugs in wartime, but became abstinent again when returned to their home-town environments (Peele & Brodsky, 1991).

IMPLICATIONS

Based on the above discussion, what can be done to help those with eating dyscontrol? In terms of treatment for the obese and/or binge eaters, the following seem to be indicated (Foreyt & Goodrick, 1994):

- Avoidance of restrictive dieting regimes. Reduction in calorie density may provide satiety, good nutrition, and minimal physiological reactivity. Regularity of eating across the day to avoid excessive hunger may enhance perceptions of self-control.
- Emphasis on social support and interpersonal skills.
- Gradual increases in enjoyable exercise (Goodrick et al., 1994).
- Use of cognitive-behavioral skills development to enhance the ability to implement a new lifestyle.
- The patient's attribution of self-blame for overeating needs to be replaced with an explanation of the biopsychosocial model, showing that symptoms are the result of a mismatch between organism and environment.

- Adjunctive pharmaceutical approaches which may alter physiological reward paths to promote prudent eating in those who manifest particular difficulty in self-control.

While it is not clear whether eating disorders can be construed as "addictions," it may be that some patients will need greater support to resist the temptations to overeat, to which they might succumb if left alone. The only weight management programs which seem to have had a long-term effect are those based on the continuous care model, which assumes a lifetime of clinical contact and scrutiny (Perri, Nezu, & Viegener, 1992).

In terms of public policy (Battle & Brownell, 1996), there are several avenues:

- Work with the food and restaurant industry to reduce the amount of calorie-dense foods, and to reduce portion sizes.
- Taxation imposed on calorie-dense foods, and subsidies for healthful foods.
- Regulation of programs in the diet industry which advocate restrictive dieting.
- Work towards greater acceptance of a diversity of body sizes, to reduce dieting behavior.

CONCLUSION

Eating, or at least the amount eaten over time for any individual, seems to be a function of environmental as well as physiological conditions. The environmental conditions include:

1. Social scrutiny to ensure prudent eating, as well as behavioral contagion associated with imprudence.
2. A plentiful food environment characterized by advertising, large displays at groceries, and a wide variety of high-calorie-dense, high-palatability foods which are easy to consume.
3. A society characterized by excessive stress, with food viewed by many as a consoling substance.
4. A society obsessed with being thin, and sharing the belief that restrictive dieting can produce thinness.

The lack of control in eating behavior which millions of Americans report experiencing takes on the appearance of what some would describe as an addiction. However, it might be more appropriately viewed as a natural mammalian response to the unnatural conditions of modern society. Short of relocating patients back to a primitive environment, "treatment" may require changing the unnatural factors involved, by altering the food supply, and by making exercise more accessible. Rather than thinking of the problem as being "within the patient," there is a need to view the entire biopsychosocial system which controls eating.

REFERENCES

Battle, E. K., & Brownell, K. D. (1996). Confronting a rising tide of eating disorders and obesity: Treatment vs. prevention and policy. *Addictive Behaviors, 21*, 755-765.

Bellisle, F. (1995). Sensory afferents and the control of eating behavior (meeting report). *Appetite, 24,* 55-56.

Bennett, W. I. (1995). Beyond overeating. *New England Journal of Medicine, 332*, 673-674.

Bennett, W. I., & Gurin, J. (1982). *The dieter's dilemma.* New York: Basic Books.

Berridge, K. C. (1991). Modulation of taste affect by hunger, caloric satiety and sensory-specific satiety in the rat. *Appetite, 16,* 103-120.

Brownell, K. D. (1991a). Personal responsibility and control over our bodies: When expectation exceeds reality. *Health Psychology, 10,* 303-310.

Brownell, K. D. (1991b). Dieting and the search for the perfect body: Where physiology and culture collide. *Behavior Therapy, 22,* 1-12.

Campfield, L. A., Smith, F. J., Rosenbaum, M., & Hirsch, J. (1996). Human eating: Evidence for a physiological basis using a modified paradigm. *Neuroscience & Biobehavioral Reviews, 20,* 133-137.

Carr, K. D., & Papadouka, V. (1994). The role of multiple opioid receptors in the potentiation of reward by food restriction. *Brain Research, 639,* 253-260.

Carr, K. D., & Simon, E. J. (1984). Potentiation of reward by hunger is opioid mediated. *Brain Research, 297,* 369-373.

Cincotta, A. H., & Meier, A. H. (1997). Bromocriptine (Ergoset) reduces body weight and improves glucose tolerance in obese diabetics. *Diabetes Care,* 19, 667-670.

Cincotta, A. H., Tozzo, E., & Scislowski, P. W. D. (1997). Bromocriptine/SKF38393 treatment ameliorates obesity and associated metabolic dysfunctions in obese (ob/ob) mice. *Life Sciences,* 61, 951-956.

Colatuoni, C., McCarthy, J., Gibbs, G., Searls, E., Alisharan, S., & Hoebel, B. G. (1997). Repeatedly restricted food access combined with highly palatable diet leads to opiate-like withdrawal symptoms during food deprivation in rats. *Society for Neuroscience Abtracts, 23,* 517.

De Vry, J., Donselaar, I., & Van Ree, J. M. (1989). Food deprivation and acquisition of intravenous cocaine self-administration in rats: Effect of naltrexone and haloperidol. *Journal of Pharmacological & Experimental Therapy, 251,* 735-740.

Drewnowski, A., Krahn, D. D., Demitrack, M. A., Nairn, K., & Gosnell, B. A. (1992). Taste responses and preferences for sweet high-fat foods: Evidence for opioid involvement. *Physiology & Behavior, 51*, 371-379.

Drewnowski, A., Kurth, C. L., & Rahaim, J. E. (1991). Taste preferences in human obesity: Environmental and familial factors. *American Journal of Clinical Nutrition, 54*, 635-641.

Dulloo, A. G., Jacquet J., & Girardier, L. (1997). Poststarvation hyperphagia and body fat overshooting in humans; a role for feedback signals from lean and fat tissues. *American Journal of Clinical Nutrition, 65*, 717-723.

Dye, L., & Blundell, J. E. (1997). Menstrual cycle and appetite control–implications for weight regulation. *Human Reproduction, 12*, 1142-1151.

Fairburn, C. G., Jones, R., Peveler, R. C., Hope, R. A., & O'Connor, M. (1993). Psychotherapy and bulimia nervosa: The longer-term effects of interpersonal psychotherapy, behavior therapy, and cognitive behavior therapy. *Archives of General Psychiatry*, 50, 419-428.

Faith, M. S., Wong, F. Y., & Allison, D. B. (1998). Demand characteristics of the research setting can influence indexes of negative affect-induced eating in obese individuals. *Obesity Research, 6*, 134-136.

Foreyt, J. P., & Goodrick, G. K. (1982). Gender and obesity. In I. Al-Issa (Ed.), *Gender and psychopathology*. New York: Academic Press.

Foreyt, J. P., & Goodrick, G. K. (1994). *Living without dieting*. New York: Warner.

Foreyt, J. P., & Goodrick, G. K. (1995). The ultimate triumph of obesity. *Lancet, 346*, 134-135.

Foreyt, J. P., & Poston, W. S. C. (1997). Diet, genetics, and obesity. *Food Technology, 51*, 70-73.

Goodrick, G. K., & Foreyt, J. P. (1991). Why treatments for obesity don't last. *Journal of the American Dietetic Association, 91*, 1243-1247.

Goodrick, G. K., Malek, J. N., & Foreyt, J. P. (1994). Exercise adherence in the obese: Self-regulated intensity. *Medicine, Exercise, Nutrition & Health, 3*, 335-338.

Greeno, C. G., & Wing, R. R. (1994). Stress-induced eating. *Psychological Bulletin, 115*, 444-464.

Grilo, C. M., Shiffman, S., & Wing, R. R. (1989). Relapse crises and coping among dieters. *Journal of Consulting & Clinical Psychology, 57*, 488-495.

Hagan, M. M., & Moss, D. E. (1991). An animal model of bulimia nervosa: Opioid sensitivity to fasting episodes. *Pharmacology, Biochemistry, & Behavior, 39*, 421-422.

Heatherton, T. F., & Baumeister, R. F. (1991). Binge eating as escape from self-awareness. *Psychological Bulletin, 110*, 86-108.

Heatherton, T. F., Polivy, J., & Herman, C. P. (1990). Restrained eating: Some current findings and speculations. *Psychology of Addictive Behaviors, 4*, 100-106.

Hoebel, B. E. (1997a). Neuroscience and appetitive behavior research: 25 years. *Appetite, 29*, 119-133.

Hoebel, B. E. (1997b). Neural systems for reinforcement and inhibition of behavior: Relevance to eating, addiction and depression. In D. Kahnerman, E. Diener & N. Schwarz (Eds.), *Understanding quality of life: Scientific perspectives on enjoyment and suffering*. Russell Sage Foundation.

International Food Policy Research Institute. (1998). *Future consumption patterns in developing countries: From rural to urban, malnutrition to obesity, sorghum to McDonald's.* (Backgrounder release). Washington, D.C.: Author.

Kayman, S., Bruvold, W., & Stern, J. (1990). Maintenance and relapse after weight-loss in women: Behavioral aspects. *American Journal of Clinical Nutrition, 52,* 800-807.

Keys, A., Brozek, J., Henschel, A., Mickelson, O., & Taylor, H. L. (1950). *The biology of human starvation.* Minneapolis: U Minnesota Press.

Klem, M. L., Wing, R. R., McGuire, M. T., Seagle, H. M., & Hill, J. O. (1997). A descriptive study of individuals successful at long-term maintenance of substantial weight loss. *American Journal of Clinical Nutrition, 66,* 239-246.

Kuczmarski, R. J., Flegal, K. M., Campbell, S. M., & Johnson, C. L. (1994). Increasing prevalence of overweight among US adults: The National Health and Nutrition Examination Surveys, 1960 to 1991. *JAMA, 272,* 205-211.

Kuehnel, R. H., & Wadden, T. A. (1994). Binge eating disorder, weight cycling, and psychopathology. *International Journal of Eating Disorders, 15,* 321-329.

Lee, A. J., Bailey, A. P. V., Yarmirr, D., O'Dea, K., & Mathews, J. D. (1994). Survival tucker: Improved diet and health indicators in an Aboriginal community. *Australian Journal of Public Health, 18,* 277-285.

Mitchell, J. E., Laine, D. E., Morley, J. E., & Levine, A. S. (1986). Naloxone but not CCK-8 may attenuate binge-eating behavior in patients with bulimia syndrome. *Biological Psychiatry, 21,* 1399-1406.

Morabia, A., Fabre, J., Chee, E., Zeger, S., Orsat, E., & Robert, A. (1989). Diet and opiate addiction: A quantitative assessment of the diet of non-institutionalized opiate addicts. *British Journal of Addiction, 84,* 173-180.

O'Dea, K. (1991). Cardiovascular disease risk factors in Australian aborigines. *Clinical & Experimental Pharmacology & Physiology, 18,* 85-88.

Peele, S., & Brodsky, A. (1991). *The truth about addiction and recovery.* New York: Fireside.

Perri, M. G., Nezu, A. M., & Viegener, B. J. (1992). *Improving the long-term management of obesity: Theory, research, and clinical guidelines.* New York: Wiley.

Poppitt, S. D., & Prentice, A. M. (1996). Energy density and its role in the control of food intake: Evidence from metabolic and community studies. *Appetite, 26,* 153-174.

Riddle, P. K. (1980). Attitudes, beliefs, behavioral intention, and behavior of women and men toward regular jogging. *Research Quarterly in Exercise & Sport, 51,* 663-674.

Ruderman, A. J. (1986). Dietary restraint: A theoretical and empirical review. *Psychological Bulletin, 99,* 247-262.

Schultz, W., Dayan, P., & Montague, P. R. (1997). A neural substrate of prediction and reward. *Science, 275,* 1593-1599.

Sjöberg, L., & Persson, L-O. (1979). A study of attempts by obese patients to regulate eating. *Addictive Behaviors, 4,* 349-359.

Stuart, R. B. (1967). Behavioral control of overeating. *Behavior Research & Therapy, 5,* 357-365.

Telch, C. F., & Agras, W. S. (1993). The effects of a very low calorie diet on binge eating. *Behavior Therapy, 24,* 177-193.

Toray, T., & Cooley, E. (1997). Weight fluctuation, bulimic symptoms, and self-efficacy for control of eating. *Journal of Psychology,* 131, 383-392.

Ward, T., Bulik, C. M., & Johnston, L. (1996). Return of the suppressed-mental control and bulimia nervosa. *Behaviour Change, 13,* 79-90.

Willenbring, M. L., Morley, J. E., Krahn, D. D., Carlson, G. A., Levine, A. S., & Shafer, R. B. (1989). Psychoneuroendocrine effects of methadone maintenance. *Psychoneuroendocrinology, 14,* 371-391.

Wilson, G. T. (1991). The addiction model of eating disorders: A critical analysis. *Advances in Behavioral Research and Therapy, 13,* 27-72.

Food as a Drug:
Conclusions

C. Keith Haddock, PhD
Walker S. Carlos Poston II, PhD

In this special collection the authors have explored the question of whether various food substances can be categorized as drugs from two overlapping angles–the potential pharmacological properties of foods and dietary supplements and the addictions model of weight and eating disorders. Although the question of whether foods act as drugs can reduce to a semantical debate over the definition of "drug" or "addiction," we believe that the authors of this series have provided useful insights into whether viewing foods as drugs is scientifically or clinically useful.

Poston et al. (Poston, Fan, Rakowski, Ericsson, Bunn, & Foreyt, 2000) provided a regulatory perspective on the issue of foods as drugs. Given the U.S. Federal Drug Administration definition of a drug (FDA, 1938), it is clear that certain naturally occurring dietary supplements (e.g., Ephedrine, St. John's Wort) meet the definition of a drug.

C. Keith Haddock and Walker S. Carlos Poston II are Assistant Professors, Department of Psychology, University of Missouri-Kansas City, and Co-Directors of Behavioral Cardiology Research, Mid America Heart Institute, St. Luke's Hospital, Kansas City, MO.

Address correspondence to: C. Keith Haddock, PhD, Department of Psychology, University of Missouri-Kansas City, Kansas City, MO 64110 (E-mail: haddockc@ umkc.edu).

The authors' work on this special series was partially supported by a faculty research grant from the University of Missouri-Kansas City and a Minority Scientist Development Award from the American Heart Association and with funds contributed by the AHA, Puerto Rico Affiliate.

[Haworth co-indexing entry note]: "Food as a Drug: Conclusions." Haddock, C. Keith, and Walker S. Carlos Poston II. Co-published simultaneously in *Drugs & Society* (The Haworth Press, Inc.) Vol. 15, No. 1/2, 1999, pp. 141-145; and: *Food as a Drug* (ed: Walker S. Carlos Poston II, and C. Keith Haddock) The Haworth Press, Inc., 2000, pp. 141-145. Single or multiple copies of this article are available for a fee from The Haworth Document Delivery Service [1-800-342-9678, 9:00 a.m. - 5:00 p.m. (EST). E-mail address: getinfo@haworthpressinc.com].

© 2000 by The Haworth Press, Inc. All rights reserved.

Furthermore, it has been argued that these substances can be characterized as foods. However, the FDA has been reticent to label any food or dietary supplement as a drug and there are no incentives in the regulatory system for manufacturers to market these substances as drugs. Poston and colleagues conclude by arguing that the distinction between synthetic drugs and food supplements is arbitrary and may hinder the medical community from harnessing the health benefits of natural products.

Chen and Volding provided a review of medicinal foods from a cross-cultural perspective (Chen & Volding, 2000). The use of various foods to improve health or cure disease has a long history in several non-Western cultures. Currently, medicinal foods are gaining popularity in Western cultures such as Germany, France, and the United States. Several herbs, such as green tea, garlic, and *Gingko biloba* have been found to have medicinal properties. For instance, *Gingko biloba* appears to improve mental information processing speed and short term memory, possibly via its effect on circulatory functioning. Although the pharmacological effects of these natural herbs are often modest compared to conventional synthetic drugs, their ability to alter physiological functioning is undeniable.

White and Reeves (2000) note that our food supply contains small quantities of many bioactive substances. Once thought immaterial to health, scientists are currently investigating the behavioral and health effects of these substances. For instance, research focused on essential oils that are found in several plant sources has demonstrated that these substances have anticarcinogenic and lipid lowering properties. White and Reeves (2000) note that bioactive substances are formed during food processing. Trans-fatty acids, for example, are formed during the hydrogenation of oils and are thought to be highly atherogenic. Thus, bioactive substances in food are likely to be significantly associated with human health. These authors also review the literature on whether the bioactive substances found in the food supply have a significant impact on mood or behavior. They conclude that the impact of nutrient and bioactive substances on mood and behavior has yet to be adequately explicated, so definitive conclusions cannot be drawn.

Haddock and Dill (2000) review the literature on whether whole foods normally eaten by Americans (e.g., carbohydrate-rich foods) have psychoactive properties and an addictive potential. Although several foods have been widely proclaimed in the scientific and popular literature as having significant effects on mood and behavior (e.g., sugar, carbohydrate-rich foods), highly controlled experiments have generally placed doubt on these claims. For instance, although sugar was once thought to produce hyperactivity in vulnerable children, placebo-controlled trials have found no relationship between sugar intake and hyperactive behavior in children. The article by Haddock and Dill reminds us that purported associations between foods and psychological functioning are subject to expectation effects.

Thus, several conclusions can be made regarding the pharmacological properties of foods. First, the U.S. government is reticent to label foods, dietary supplements, or herbs as drugs despite potential medicinal properties of these substances. Second, the food substances that have demonstrated medicinal qualities are either not typically consumed or are not consumed in quantities to produce a significant pharmacological effect in the typical American diet unless they are taken via supplementation. Finally, the whole foods typically consumed in the American diet generally have not been found to have significant psychopharmacological or addictive properties.

Given the paucity of evidence that foods found in the dietary matrix are addictive, it is not surprising that Stein and colleagues (Stein, O'Byrne, Suminski, & Haddock, 2000), Haddock and Dill (2000), Wilson (2000), and Goodrick (2000) conclude that the addictions model of obesity and eating disorders does not provide a compelling model for these serious disorders. Stein and colleagues (Stein et al., 2000) reviewed the literature on the etiology and treatment of obesity and conclude that the central tenants of the addictions model lack empirical support. Alternatively, the most promising theories of both the increasing prevalence of obesity and obesity treatment involve environmental or public health approaches, not models that view the controlling factors for obesity as residing "within the skin" of the patient. Haddock and Dill (2000) argued that the central tenet of the addictions model of obesity, that certain food substances that are plentiful in the American diet have significant psychoactive properties and are addictive, lacks sufficient support. Furthermore, they noted that the evidence that a specific "carbohydrate craving" disorder supports the addictions model in a subpopulation of obese individuals is lacking. Both Wilson (2000) and Goodrick (2000) suggest that although eating disorders and obesity have some characteristics similar to substance abuse and dependence, the overlap is quite weak. For example, neither tolerance for nor withdrawal from whole foods found in the American diet have been demonstrated.

Goodrick (2000) proposes that an alternative explanation to the addictions model of the seemingly compulsive nature of eating among many individuals is that they are having a normal response to an abnormal environment. That is, we have been genetically programmed to gather and consume foods (i.e., in case of famine) and to conserve energy. Given (1) a plentiful supply of calorically-dense and highly palatable foods, (2) a decreasing need to be physically active, and (3) a society obsessed with being thin, it is not surprising that we eat compulsively and then experience negative emotional reactions to our eating. Goodrick concludes that the etiology of excessive dietary intake is an environment that is incompatible with our evolutionary heritage.

In conclusion, there is little doubt that certain naturally-occurring food substances impact human health analogous to the effects found for many synthetic drugs. Despite this, regulatory agencies in the United States appear reticent to classify any food substances as drugs. The parallel between foods and drugs becomes weak, however, when one juxtaposes the effects of foods with that of psychoactive or addictive drugs. Thus, eating-related disorders such as obesity and bulimia nervosa are not likely the result of a drug-like dependence on certain foods. Rather, these eating disorders are likely the result of potent environmental factors that lead to unhealthy dietary practices.

REFERENCES

Chen, C. H., & Volding, D. C. (2000). Medicinal foods: Cross cultural perspectives. In Poston, W. S. C. & Haddock, C. K. (Eds.), *Food as a drug* (pp. 49-64). New York, NY: The Haworth Press, Inc.

Goodrick, G. K. (2000). Inability to control eating: Addiction to food or normal response to an abnormal environment? In Poston, W. S. C. & Haddock, C. K. (Eds.), *Food as a drug* (pp. 123-140). New York, NY: The Haworth Press, Inc.

Haddock, C. K., & Dill, P. L. (2000). The effects of food on mood and behavior: Implications for the addictions model of obesity. In Poston, W. S. C. & Haddock, C. K. (Eds.), *Food as a drug* (pp. 17-47). New York, NY: The Haworth Press, Inc.

Poston, W. S. C., Fan, L., Rakowski, R., Ericsson, M., Bunn, C. C., & Foreyt, J. P. (2000). Legal and regulatory perspectives on dietary substances. In Poston, W. S. C. & Haddock, C. K. (Eds.), *Food as a drug* (pp. 65-85). New York, NY: The Haworth Press, Inc.

Stein, R. J., O'Byrne, K. K., Suminski, R. R., & Haddock, C. K. (2000). Etiology and treatment of obesity in adults and children: Implications for the addiction model. In Poston, W. S. C. & Haddock, C. K. (Eds.), *Food as a drug* (pp. 103-121). New York, NY: The Haworth Press, Inc.

White, J. V., & Reeves, R. S. (2000). Pharmacological properties of foods and nutrients. In Poston, W. S. C. & Haddock, C. K. (Eds.), *Food as a drug* (pp. 1-16). New York, NY: The Haworth Press, Inc.

Wilson, G. T. (2000). Eating disorders and addiction. In Poston, W. S. C. & Haddock, C. K. (Eds.), *Food as a drug* (pp. 87-101). New York, NY: The Haworth Press, Inc.

Index

5-HT. *See also* Serotonin
    enzymes and, 37
    mood regulation and, 35-36
    production of, 36
5-HT biosynthesis
    carbohydrate consumption and, 39
    diet and, 39
    enzymes and, 36
    tryptophan and, 36-37

Aboriginal Australians, obesity and,
    lifestyle influence on, 135
Abstinence
    addiction model and, 91,115
    counterindicated for binge eating,
      91-92
    food addiction therapy and, 18
    obesity management and, 103-104
    obesity treatment, 114
Addiction
    definition, 88,124,141
    eating disorders as, weight
      management programs and,
      136
    hallmark of, 132-133
    steps for, 132
Addictions model
    12-step approach called for in, 91
    abstinence and, 91
    alternative explanation, normal
      response to abnormal
      environment, 144
    carbohydrate consumption and,
      unsupported by literature, 39
    eating disorders and, 88,143
    food addictions, example of
      treatments for obesity,
      113-114
    foods acting as drugs under, 141
    obese binge eaters and, 91

obesity and, 17,103-104,124-125,
    143
    dietary intake and, 115
    problems with, 124-125
    premises of, 115
    psychoactive substances, food
      viewed as, 20
    treatment implications for, 91-92
    treatments based on, efficacy of,
      115
Addictive disorders, psychoactive
    substances and, 21
Addictive personality, for foods, no
    evidence for, 125
ADHD. *See* Attention Deficit
    Hyperactivity Disorder
    (ADHD)
Alcohol
    drug dependence disorder and, 18
    effects differ from food, 41
    psychoactive effects of, compared
      with foods, 17
Alcohol problems. *See* Substance
    abuse
Alcoholism
    addiction model and, 106
    eating disorders and, 95-96
    obesity similiar to, 106
Allergic tension-fatigue syndrome,
    food allergies and, 22
Allicin, constituent of garlic, 55-56
Allium (genus) plants, effects of, 4-5
Allium sativum (garlic). *See also*
    Garlic
    history of use, 54-55
Alzheimer's disease, *Ginkgo biloba*
    extract (GBE) and, 58
Amino acids. *See also* Dietary
    supplements
    dietary supplement, 67

© 2000 by The Haworth Press, Inc. All rights reserved.

147

use in US, 66-67
Dietary Supplement Health and
    Education Act of 1994 and,
    71
regulation of brain
    neurotransmission and, 11
Anorexia nervosa
    eating disorder, 87
    substance abuse
        association with, 93-94
        lifetime rates and, 92
Anorexia nervosa patients, substance
    abuse in families of, 96
Anti-bacterial effect, of garlic, 55-56
Anti-cancer activities, of garlic, 55
Anti-cholesterolemic activity, tea
    extract and, 52
Anti-inflammatory properties
    of ginger, 56
    phenolic compounds and, 4
Anticarcinogenic properties
    of *Allium* plants, 4-5
    of essential oils, 4,142
    of plant constituents, similar to
        synthetic antioxidants, 5
Antidepressant properties, St. John's
    Wort, 59-60,76
Antimutagenic properties, of *Allium*
    plants, 4-5
Antinauseant properties, of ginger, 56
Antioxidant mechanisms, tea extract,
    plasma lipid profile
    improvement and, 52
Antioxidant properties
    of phenolic compounds, 4
    of plant constituents, similar to
        synthetic antioxidants, 5
Antiseptic potentials, of garlic, 55
Antispasmodic properties, of ginger,
    56
Antitumor properties, of flavones, 4
Antiviral properties, St. John's Wort,
    60
Appetite
    neuroscience and, research,
        131-132

psychophysical conditions of, 133
Appetite stimulation, food restriction
    and, 131
Appetite suppressant mediation,
    demand, 125
Arthritis, ginger and, 57
Aspirin senstivity
    food additives and, 23
    salicylate-free diet and, 23
Attention Deficit Hyperactivity
    Disorder (ADHD), sugar and,
    21

BED. *See* Binge Eating Disorder
    (BED)
Bee pollen, as dietary supplement, 67
Behavioral disorders, childhood, diet
    and, no evidence for, 35
Behavioral influences
    of bioactive substances, 2
    on children, food, 22-23
Behavioral modification
    bioactive substances and, 142
    foods and, 21,142-143
    obesity treatment, 111-112
        pharmacological interventions
            and, 112
    weight loss programs and, clinical
        trials of, 111-112
Behavioral programs, obesity
    treatment
    activity level increase, 111
    components of, 111
    eating habits modification, 111
    efficacy of, 115
Behavioral sensitization phase, of
    addiction, 132
Binge eating
    bulimic patients and, 89-90
    case illustration of, 90
    cognitive-behavioral therapy
        (CBT), effective treatment,
        98
    compulsive overeating, triggers,
        130-131
    control loss, 88

drug dependence compared with, 130-131
food addiction model and, 18
implications for treatment, 135-136
mood alteration and, 18
nondieting treatments and, 114
obesity and, 108,113-114,115
opiate antagonists, used to reduce, 132
opiates and, 130
rationale for, 129
weight control and, 90-91
women, control and, 133-134
Binge Eating Disorder (BED), eating disorder, 88
Bioactive peptides
curing of meat and, 5
digestion of casein and, 5
Bioactive substances
animal products, purported health attributes of, 5
classes of, 2-7
effects of, 2-7
in food, 2,142
food processing and, 2,5-6,142
hydrolysis of food proteins, effects of, 6
impact on mood, problems with assessment of, 7
multifunctional roles of, 2
ocurrence of, 2
plant products
glucosinolates, 3-4
purported health attributes of, 3-5
production of, in vivo, 2
Biopsychosocial model, explanation as treatment, self-blame replaced by, 135
Biopsychosocial system, eating behavior and, 137
Blood-brain barrier
neurotransmitter synthesis and, 36
role in tryptophan synthesis, 37
Blood-glucose levels
insulin level and, 28

sugar's mechanism, hyperactivity and, 28
Blood pressure, caffeine intake and, 12
Blood serum cholesterol levels
tea consumption and, studies of, 52
tea extract and, 52
Blood sugar levels. *See also* Blood-glucose levels
brain reaction to, 28
rapid decline in, behavioral symptoms and, 28
BMI. *See* Body Mass Index (BMI)
Body image, dissatisfaction and, 126-127
Body Mass Index (BMI), obesity and, 104
Body shape
attitudes toward, 95-96
eating disorders and, 91,92
Body sizes, acceptance of diversity in, 136
Body weight
attitudes toward, 95-96
eating disorders and, 91,92
Boredom, overeating rationale, 129
Botanicals, Dietary Supplement Health and Education Act of 1994 and, 71
Brassica vegetable family, cancer prevention and, 3-4
Bulimia nervosa
alcohol problems of parents, risk factor for, 96
cognitive-behavioral therapy (CBT), effective treatment, 98
eating disorder, 87
environmental factors of, 144
etiology, 144
serotonin activity reduction in women with, 11
study with carbohydrate binge in, 88-89
substance abuse
association with, 93-95
lifetime rates and, 92

Bulimia nervosa patients
  binge eating and, 89-90
  meals of, 89
  situational control and, 134
  substance abuse in families of, 96

Caffeine. *See also* Coffee
  accumulation in vivo, 21
  interaction with synaptic
      macromolecules, 21
  physiologic function effects, 12
Caloric consumption, perception of
      pain and, 8
Calorie-dense foods
  in food environment, obesity and,
      124
  taxation on, as public policy
      avenue, 136
Calories
  consumption increase, in
      premenstrual women, 7-8
  consumption of, obesity and, 124
Camellia sinensis, tea as product of,
      51
Cancer incidence, green tea
      consumption and, 52
Cancer prevention. *See also*
      Anticarcinogenic properties
  bioactive substances, plant products
      and, 3-5
  Brassica vegetable family and, 3-4
  soybean products and, 53
Carbohydrate binge, study with
      bulimia nervosa patients,
      88-89
Carbohydrate consumption
  5-HT biosynthesis and, 39-40
  effects of, 8-9
  mood and, 8-9
  placebo effects and, 89
  protein and, 39-40
  serotonergic neurotransmission,
      drugs that increase and, 40
  serotonin release and, 9-10
  tryptophan/LNAA ratio alteration
      and, 39

Carbohydrate craving
  addictions model, lack of support
      for, 143
  etiology of, 40
  evidence lacking, 87
  obesity and, 39,40
    5-HT biosynthesis and, 40-41
    gender difference in, 40
    mood unimproved after, 41
    problems with model, 40-41
Carbohydrate-rich foods
  addictive potential of, 142-143
  psychoactive properties of, 142-143
Carbohydrates. *See also* Nutrients
  binge eating and, 108
  childhood obesity and, 113-114
  mood regulation and, 88
  refined
    blood-glucose levels and, 28
    as trigger for food addiction, 18
  tryptophan and, 88
Cardiovascular diseases
  green tea consumption and, 52-53
  protection against
    garlic, 55
    green tea, 52-53
  soybean products and, 53
    hypocholesterolemic protective
      effects of, 54
Cardiovascular effects, of garlic
  hypertension treatment and, 55
  multiple, 55
CBT. *See* Cognitive-behavioral
      therapy (CBT)
Challenge experiment, diet-behavior
      research, recommended for,
      33
Chemical dependency. *See also*
      Addiction
  defining characteristics of, 88
Chemopreventive effects, of
      glucosinolates, 3-4
Chicken extract (BEC)
  chicken soup and folklore, 12-13
  effects of, 12-13
Chicken soup. *See* Chicken extract

Childhood obesity
    addiction model, plausibility of, 113
    behavioral programs for, promising
        results of, 111
    carbohydrates and, 113-114
    Hispanic-American children and, 104
    Native-American children and, 104
    risks of, 104-105
    treatment approaches to, 110-115
Chocolate
    bioactive substances of, 11
    food cravings and, 11
    sensory attributes of, 11
Circulatory functioning, *Gingko
        biloba* and, 142
Coffee. *See also* Caffeine
    effects of, 12
    mood improvement and, 11-12
Cognitive-behavior skills, as
        treatment, use of, 135
Cognitive-behavioral therapy (CBT)
    binge eating and, 90
        effective treatment for, 98
    bulimia nervosa, effective
        treatment for, 98
    eating disorders, efficacy for, 91-92
Cognitive-behavioral treatment (CBT).
        See Cognitive-behavioral
        therapy (CBT)
Cognitive functioning, *Gingko biloba*
        and, 142
Cognitive modification, obesity
        treatment and, 111-112
Compulsive eating, in overweight
        individuals, 18
Consumer information, Dietary
        Supplement Health and
        Education Act of 1994 and, 72
Consumers
    dietary supplements and, 68-69
        adverse medication interaction
            and, 80
        health care providers
            uninformed of use, 80
        information sources, 80
    profile of, 68-69

Consumption patterns
    changing, 134-135
    Minjilang Project, 135
Control. *See also* Eating control
    actual vs perceived, 126,127
    cognitive processes and, 127
    cultural assumptions regarding, 126
    exercise and, 127
    loss of
        addiction and, 132-133
        binge eating and, 88
    obesity and, 125,126
    perception of, 128-129
    physiological processes and, 127
    willpower and, 126
Correlational studies, diet-behavior
        research and, 31-32
Craving phase, of addiction, 132
Cravings
    addiction model and, 18
    as biochemical result, no
        compelling evidence for, 88
    carbohydrate
        mood regulation and, 39
        obese individuals and, 40
    eating disorders and, 88
    sweet, associated with opium
        addiction, 130
    symptom of obesity, 125
Cultural environment, effects on
        obesity, 109-110
Cultural influences, weight
        management programs and,
        128
Culture, obesity and, 109-110
Curcumin, polyphenolic compound, 4
Cyclamates. *See also* Food additives
    in artificial sweeteners, 23

Depression
    dietary supplements and, 73
    food and, 22
    St. John's Wort and, 59-60
Devices, regulation of, Food and Drug
        Modernization Act of 1997
        and, 72

Diabetes, non-insulin dependent,
    obesity and, 105
Diet
  high carbohydrate
    behavior alteration and, 38
    mood alteration and, 38,39
    tryptophan levels and, 38
  hyperactivity and, 26-27
  recommended, 14
Diet-behavior research
  early
    causal claims based on
      correlational data, 31
    expectancy biases, 31
    placebo group lack, 31
    sampling problems, 31
    uncontrolled studies, 31
  link, double-blind procedures, 35
    disappearance of, 34-35
  methodological flaws in, 31-34
  study design for, 32-33
Diet composition, effects of, 10
Diet industry, regulation needed, 136
Diet patterns, change, obesity
    treatment and, 111-112
Dietary intake
  obesity and, 106,115
  obesity factor, 107-108
  research on, 107-108
Dietary protein, tryptophan synthesis,
    blood-brain barrier and, 37
Dietary restriction
  addiction model and, 91
  counterindications for, 91
Dietary substances, Dietary Supplement
    Health and Education Act of
    1994 and, 71
Dietary Suplement Health and
    Education Act of 1994,
    evidence required by, 78
Dietary Supplement Health and
    Education Act of 1994
  burden of proof and, 71
  dietary supplement definition, 67
  dietary supplement regulation,
    guidance for, 69

dietary supplements and, 65-66
  efficacy and, 71
  FDA, burden of proof, 73
  history of, 69-70
  safety and, 71
  summary of, 71-72
Dietary supplement manufacturers
  new drug application (NDA)
    patents not possible, 81-82
    process and, 80
  nomenclature consistency and, 81
  quality standards and, 80-81
  research, no incentive for, 80
Dietary supplement safety
  efficacy, need for examination of,
    81
  health claims, need for examination
    of, 81
  safety, need for examination of, 81
Dietary supplements. *See also*
    Nutritional supplements
  as alternative method of health
    care, 68
  benefits reported
    disease intervention, 68
    energy improvement, 68
  case studies, 74-77
  consumer, typical, 68-69
  definitions, 66
    Dietary Supplement Health and
      Education Act of 1994, 67,71
    FDA requirements regarding,
      70-71
  disease prevention and, 73
  distinguished from drugs, 82
    health claims and, 73-74
    unclear, 73
  economic impact of, 69
  efficacy of
    Dietary Supplement Health and
      Education Act of 1994 and, 71
    regulatory agencies and, 69
  Ephedrine, drug definition and, 141
  information regarding, consumers',
    80
  legal status of, 69-71

legislation pertaining to, 65-66
   Dietary Supplement Health and
      Education Act, 65-66
market for, 65
oversight recommendations for, 82
pharmacological properties of, 141
prevalence of, 65,66-67
principle of proportionality
      suggested for, 82
quality of
   impact of legislation on, 74
   regulatory agencies and, 69
regulatory approach
   agencies and, 69
   limitations of, 78-79
regulatory standards
   changes to improve, 66
   dangers of current, 66
safety of
   burden of proof and, 72
   Dietary Supplement Health and
      Education Act of 1994 and, 71
   impact of legislation on, 74
   problems, FDA and, 77
   regulatory agencies and, 69
St. John's Wort, drug definition
     and, 141
studies, reasons for taking, 67,68
survey data regarding, 68
use, 65
   impact of legislation on, 74
   treatment of health problems,
     67-68
   typical, 67-68
   widespread, 69
Dietary tryptophan, depression and, 22
Dieters dilemma, description of, 125
Dieting, restrictive
control assumptions and, 126-127
physiological correlates of, 128
psychological correlates of, 128
results of, 128
Diets
   as cures for diseases, 18
   as cures for psychological
     problems, 18

food supply, role in obesity,
     107-108
obese vs lean individuals, 107-108
Disease prevention
   dietary supplement use and, 67
   dietary supplements and, 73
Disease treatment, dietary
     supplements and, 73
Diseases
   modulators of, 1-2
   nutrients as modulators of, 1
   obesity and, 105
Dopamine reward theory, eating
     behavior and, 132
Double-blind placebo controlled
     experiment, diet-behavior
     research, recommended for, 33
Drug addictions
   alcohol and, 19
   dependencies and, 19-20
   nicotine and, 19
   psychoactive properties of abused
     substance and, 20
Drug Amendments, response to
     thalidomide tragedy, 70
Drug companies, St. John's Wort and,
     78
Drug dependence
   criteria of, 19,20
   diagnostic criteria of, 19
Drugs
   definition, 141
   distinguished from supplements,
     82, 142
     health claims and, 73-74
     unclear, 73
   federal regulation of, 69-71
   food substances characterized as,
     141
   as foods, 144
   interstate commerce requirements
     for, 70
   obesity management, 112-113
   regulation of, Food and Drug
     Modernization Act of 1997
     and, 72

Eating
    decision, influences on, 133-134
    environmental conditions and,
        136-137
Eating behaviors
    dopamine reward theory and, 132
    natural response vs addiction,
        136-137
    physiological processes result in,
        131-132
    rituals and, 128
    treatment for
        biopsychosocial system and, 137
        changing unnatural factors, 137
        exercise and, 137
        food supply alteration, 137
Eating control
    cultural translocation and, 133
    dieting and, 126-127
    factors involved in, 133
    loss of
        abnormal situation and, 125
        as addiction, no evidence for,
            125
        explanation of, 125
        public health interventions and,
            125
        symptom of obesity, 124-125
    obesity symptoms and, 125
    perception of, 128-129
    physiological evidence and, 130
    restrictive diets, 130
        results of, 128
    willpower and, 126-127
Eating Disorder Examination
        (EDE-Q), eating disorder
        assessment technique, 98
Eating disorders
    addictions model of, 88,143
        problems with, 88-91
    alcoholism and, 95-96
    attributed to food addiction, pitfalls
        with, 19-20
    biobehavioral explanations for
        features, 87
    as chemical disorders, 20

patient concerns, 92
    seeking treatment for, 93
    substance abuse
        accelerated by, 97
        association with, 92-96,95,97
            reciprocal reinforcement
                theory of, 97
        dependence distinguished from,
            87
        distinguished from, 87,143-144
        families of patients with, 96
        mechanisms linking, 97
        resemblance to, 88
        similarities, 143-144
    substance abuse screening
        recommended, 97-98
Eating Disorders Not Otherwise
        Specified (EDNOS), eating
        disorder, 87-88
Eating dyscontrol. *See* Binge eating;
        Eating control; Obesity
EC. *See* Ephedrine, and caffeine (EC)
Echinacea
    extended use of, harmful side
        effects, 60
    immune-stimulation effects of, 59
    medicinal qualities, 51
    uses of, 59
Echinacea angustifolia. *See* Echinacea
Echinacea purpurea. *See also*
        Echinacea therapeutic
        effects, belief in, 58
EDNOS. *See* Eating Disorders Not
        Otherwise Specified
        (EDNOS)
Elaidic acid, effects of, 6
Energy, dietary supplement use and,
        67
Energy expenditure
    increase of, obesity treatment and,
        111-112
    obesity and, 106
Environment
    abnormal, normal response to, 144
    cultural, effects on obesity, 109-110
    obesity and, 109-110,115

Environmental approaches, obesity
　　treatment and, 143
Environmental conditions
　　food environment characterization,
　　　136
　　social scrutiny and, 136
　　society characterization, 136
Enzymatic digestion, industrial
　　bioactive substances as result of, 2
　　food processing activities and, 2
Enzymes
　　addiction to food, biologic activity
　　　and, 7
　　addiction to food, potential for
　　　deterioration and, 7
Ephedra (Ma Huang)
　　as dietary supplement, 67
　　weight loss and, 75
Ephedrine
　　adverse effects, FDA reports of, 77
　　and caffeine (EC)
　　　safety of, 75
　　　studies of, 75
　　　weight loss and, 75
　　dietary supplement, 66
　　as drug, 141
　　efficacy of, 77
　　as food, 142
　　safety of, 77
Ephedrine and caffeine (EC)
　　long-term administration, effects,
　　　75-76
　　side effects, 75-76
Epidemiological data, serum cholesterol
　　levels, mood and, 9
Epidemiological studies
　　cancer prevention, Brassica
　　　vegetable family and, 3
　　eating disorders, substance abuse
　　　association, 93-95
　　PAHs and, 6
Ergogenic aids, dietary supplement
　　use and, 67
Ergogenic claims, sassafras, 74-75
Essential oils. *See also* Terpenes
　　bioactive substances, 142

Exercise
　　lack of
　　　control and, 127
　　　obesity and, 124,127
　　as treatment, increase of, 135
Exercise behavior, physiological
　　influence on, 127
Expectancy biases, diet-behavior
　　research and, 31
Expectancy effects
　　diet-behavior research and, 32-33
　　food additives, problem behavior
　　　and, 34
　　K-P diet and, 27
　　problem behavior, sugar and, 34
Expectation effects. *See also*
　　　Expectancy effects
　　food-mood associations and, 143
Extranutritional components. *See also*
　　　Bioactive substances in food, 2

Fat. *See* Nutrients
Fat consumption
　　effects of, change during day, 8-9
　　mood and, 8-9
Fatigue, ergogenic product sales and,
　　67
FDA. *See* Food and Drug
　　　Administration (FDA)
Federal Food, Drug, and Cosmetic
　　　Act, pharmaceutical
　　　regulation and, 70
Feingold
　　Kaiser-Permanente (K-P) diet,
　　　23-24
　　theories of, 23-25
Feingold Diet. *See also*
　　　Kaiser-Permanente (K-P)
　　　diet
　　persistance of, 34
Feingold K-P diet. *See*
　　　Kaiser-Permanente (K-P)
　　　diet
Fermented soybean products,
　　examples, 53
Fiber. *See* Nutrients

Flavones, antioxidative properties of, 4

Flavonoids
effects of, 4
Ginkgo biloba extract and, 57
in tea, 12

Folklore Medicines, nomenclature, Canadian model, 81

Food acceptance
heating and, 6
prolonged storage and, 6

Food addictions
abstinence, of refined carbohydrates, 18
animal model of, 131-132
binge eating as characteristic of, 113-114
characterization of, 113-114
childhood formation of, 113-114
definition of, 18
etiology of, 18
genetic susceptibility and, 18
seriousness of, 18-19
therapeutic regimen for, 18

Food addictions model. *See also* Addictions model
for obesity, 18
pitfalls with, 19-20

Food-additive-free diet, Kaiser-Permanente (K-P) diet, effects of, 23-24

Food additives
ADHD and, 21
behavior and
change in children, anecdotal reports, 22
methodological flaws in research, 31
problem
as cause of, 24
expectancy effects and, 34
link unsubstantiated, 34
ginger root, 56
hyperactive behavior, 27
in children
doubts of causality of, 31

expectancy effects and, 34
increase, 22-23
popular belief in link persists, 34

Food allergies. *See also* Food dye allergy; Food sensitivities
allergic tension-fatigue syndrome and, 22

Food and Drug Act of 1906
pharmaceutical regulation and, 70
Sherley Amendment to, 70

Food and Drug Administration (FDA)
agency constraints, 78
authority of, 70,72,73
burden of proof and, 72,73
dietary supplements
definition, 67
implications of use, 66
drugs, definition of, 141
health claims, 81
drugs vs dietary supplements, 73-74
label disclaimer and, 72

Food and Drug Modernization Act of 1997
dietary supplements and, 65-66
regulation guidance, 69
evidence required by, 78
food labeling and, 73
history of, 69-70
summary, 72-73

Food colorings. *See also* Food additives
hyperactive behavior increase, in children, 22-23

Food components. *See also* Bioactive substances; Extranutritional components
accumulation in vivo, 21
interaction with synaptic macromolecules, 21
terms defined, 2,3

Food consumption
mood and, 8
premenstrual women, increase in, 7-8

timing of, cognitive performance
and, 8
Food cravings
chocolate, 11
pizza, 11
Food deprivation
dopamine reward theory and, 132
reward value of food increased by,
131
sleep deprivation, comparison,
89-90
Food dye allergy. *See also* Food
allergies
hyperactivity and, 24
Food environment
characterization of, 136
importance of, 134
Food flavorings. *See* Food additives
Food industry, calorie-dense foods,
reduce amount of, as public
policy avenue, 136
Food preservation procedures, PAHs
and, 6
Food processing
bioactive substances and, 142
heating, results of, 6
PAHs and, 6
prevalence of, 5-6
results of commonly used methods,
6
Food restriction
appetite stimulation and, 131
dopamine reward theory and, 132
Food sensitivities. *See also* Food
allergies
hyperactive behavior and, 24-25
testing for, problems with, 26-27
Food substances
behavior effects of, 41
as drugs, 141
effects, differ from psychoactive
drugs, 41
effects on human health, 144
mood effects of, 41
Food supplements, distinguished from
drugs, 142

Food supply
bioactive substances in, 142
disease modulators in, 1-2
health modulators in, 1-2
Foods. *See also* Food components
addictive properties of, not found,
143
behavior alteration and, 20
biological consequences of, 89-90
as consoling, 136
distinguished from psychoactive
substance, 21
as drugs, 88,141,144
historical claims of, 18
labels and, 143
regulatory perspective on, 141
environment of abundant, 130
health claims, restrictions for,
73-74
heating, results of, 6
impact on mood, 14
medicinal qualities of, quantities
required for, 143
medicinal uses of
popularity of, 60
traditions of, 49-50
worldwide sales of, 60
mood regulation and, 20,89
pharmacological properties of,
1-16,141
conclusions regarding, 143
processing, appetite maximized,
130
psychoactive effects of, 17,21-22
compared with psychoactive
drugs, 17
psychoactive substance, not
considered as, 21-22
as psychoactive substances,
addictions model and, 20
psychopharmacological properties
of, not found, 143
regulation of, Food and Drug
Modernization Act of 1997
and, 72-73
tolerance not demonstrated, 87

withdrawal not demonstrated, 87
FRG. *See* Functional reactive
        hypoglycemia (FRG)
Functional reactive hypoglycemia
        (FRG)
    blood-glucose levels and, 28-29
    hyperactivity relationship, 28-29
Fungicidal properties, of garlic, 55-56
Fungistatic activities, of garlic, 55-56

Garlic. *See also Allium sativum*
        (garlic)
    allicin constituent of, 55-56
    antiseptic potentials of, 55
    cardiovascular effects of, 55
    circulatory functioning and, 60
    health-promoting effects of, 55
    history of use, 54
    immune-stimulating properties of,
        55-56
    medicinal qualities, 49,51,142
    use of, 54-55
Genetics, obesity factor, 107
Genistein, anti-carcinogen, 53
German Commission E system
    drugs and supplements, double
        standard for, 82
    FDA and, 81
Ginger. *See also Zingiber officinale*
        (ginger)
    anti-inflammatory properties of,
        56,57
    as antidote to food poisoning, 56
    circulatory functioning and, 60
    historical traditions of, 56
    medicinal qualities, 49,51,56-57
    motion sickness remedy, 56-57
        inconclusive, 557
    motion sickness study
        with dimenhydrinate, 56
        with placebo, 56
    powdered, motion sickness remedy,
        56
Gingerbread, evolution of, 56
Ginkgo biloba extract (GBE)
    Alzheimer's disease and, 58

congnitive deficits and, 57,58
effects of, 57
flavonoids isolated from, 57
prescribed in Europe, for cognitive
        deficits, 57
Ginkgo biloba (ginkgo tree)
    adverse side effects of, 60,61
    Chinese traditional medicine and, 57
    circulatory functioning and, 60
    extract (*See Ginkgo biloba* extract
        (GBE))
    medicinal qualities, 49,51,142
    seeds, remedy for ailments, 57
Ginseng
    adverse side effects of, 60
    Chinese pharmacology and, 58
    circulatory functioning and, 60
    as dietary supplement, 67
    health-promoting qualities of,
        scientific investigation and,
        59
    medicinal qualities, 51,58-59
        belief in, 58
    modern beliefs about, 59
Glandular products. *See* Tissue
        extracts
Glucosinolates, cancer prevention and,
        3-4
Green tea
    cancer incidence and, 52
    cardiovascular disease, protective
        action against, 52-53
    history of, 51
    medicinal qualities, 49,51,142
    phenolic component of, 4
Guarana (caffeine), as dietary
        supplement, 67

Haptens, in food additives, 23
Health
    modulators of, 1-2
    nutrients as modulators of, 1
Health claims
    Canadian model for, 81
    distinction between drug and
        dietary supplements, 73

German model for, 81
new drug application (NDA) and, 73-74
Health enhancement, dietary supplement use and, 67
Health problems, dietary supplements used to treat, 68
Healthful foods, subsidies of, as public policy avenue, 136
Heart disease. *See also* Cardiovascular diseases
 risk factors, reduction through tea, 52-53
Hepatotoxicity, echinacea and, 60
Herbal medicinals
 drug interactions and, 60
 risks of side effects, 60
 scientific questions regarding, 61
 worldwide sales of, 60
Herbal preparations. *See also* Dietary supplements; Herbal medicinals
 dietary supplement, use in US, 66-67
 historical, 50-51
 trial and error in developing, 50-51
Herbals, historical, 50-51
Herbs
 Dietary Supplement Health and Education Act of 1994 and, 71
 as drugs, labels and, 143
Heroin addiction, obesity similiar to, 106
Hispanic-American children, obesity among, 104
HOD Test. *See* Hoffer-Osmond Diagnostic (HOD) Test
Hoffer-Osmond Diagnostic (HOD) Test, maladaptive behaviors assessed by, 30
Hormones, blood-glucose levels and, 28
Hyperactivity. *See also* Hyperkinesis
 in children, sugar and, 143
 diet and, 26-27

studies of, 22
 food additives and, 22-23,25-26,27
 food dye allergy and, 24
 food sensitivities and, support for, 24-25
 functional reactive hypoglycemia (FRG), blood-glucose levels and, 28-29
 K-P diet and, 23
 sugar association with, 29
 expectation effects of, 143
 link dubious, 33-34
 studies with children, 29-30
Hypericin, St. John's Wort extract, safety of. *See* St. John's Wort
Hypericum perforatum. See St. John's Wort; St. John's wort
Hyperkinesis. *See also* Hyperactivity
 behavioral problems characteristic of
 double-blind study of, 25
 judgments regarding, 25
 food additives and, 23
Hyperphagia, eating control and, 130
Hypertension treatment, garlic and, 55
Hypocholesterolemic effects, soybean products, against cardiovascular disease, 54
Hypoglycemia
 influence on aggressive behavior and
 Hoffer-Osmond Diagnostic (HOD)Test, 30
 study of prision population, 30
 sucrose consumption and, 21
Hypolipemic mechanisms, tea extract, plasma lipid profile improvement and, 52

Immune-stimulation, echinacea and, 59
Immuniologic influences, of bioactive substances, 2
Indoles, cancer prevention and, 3-4
Intradermal titration method, food allergy testing and, 26-27
Isoflavones. *See also* Genistein

genistein, soybean constituent, 53
Isoflavonoids, effects of, 4

Kaiser-Permanente (K-P) diet
    effects of, 23-24
    efficacy unsupported, 27
    food-additive free, 23-24

Labels
    Dietary Supplement Health and
        Education Act of 1994 and,
        71-72
    Food and Drug Modernization Act
        of 1997 and, 73
    foods as drugs, US government
        reticence regarding, 143
    health claims and, 79
    requirements of, 71-72
    standardized, 71-72
Labor-saving devices, obesity and,
    109-110
Large neutral amino acid (LNAA)
    tryptophan. *See* Tryptophan
Learning disabilities
    functional reactive hypoglycemia
        (FRG), blood-glucose levels
        and, 28-29
    K-P diet and, 23
Legislation, problems with current,
    77-78
Lipid lowering properties
    of *Allium* plants, 4-5
    essential oils and, 4,142
    of flavonoids, 4
    of isoflavonoids, 4
LNAA. *See* Tryptophan

Ma Huang (ephedra). *See* Ephedra
    (Ma Huang)
Macronutrients
    intake of, role in obesity, 108
    mood and, 73

Maillard reaction products (MRPs),
    activity caused by, 6
MAOI. *See* Monoamine oxidase
    inhibitor (MAOI)
Medical problems, obesity and, 104-105
Medicinal foods
    cross-cultural perspective on, 142
    traditions of, 49
Medicinal herbs
    historical recordings of, 50-51
    history of, 49-50,50-51
Memory, *Ginkgo biloba* extract and,
    58
Methodological issues, diet-behavior
    research and, 31-34
Methylphenidate
    Attention Deficit Disorder and, 35
    placebo substituted for, 35
Minerals. *See also* Dietary
        supplements; Nutrients
    dietary supplement, use in US,
        66-67
    Dietary Supplement Health and
        Education Act of 1994 and,
        71
Minjilang Project, food environment
    and, 135
Monoamine oxidase inhibitor (MAOI),
    St. John's Wort as, 79
Mood, impact of bioactive substances
    on, problems with
    assessment of, 7
Mood alteration. *See also* Negative
        emotions
    bioactive substances and, 142
    carbohydrate craving and, 39
    foods and, 21,142-143
    St. John's Wort and, 59
Motion sickness, ginger as remedy for,
    56
MRPs. *See* Maillard reaction products
    (MRPs)
Musculoskeletal disorders, ginger and,
    57
Mutagenic substances, from animal
    products, 5

N-nitroso compounds, inhibition of
 formation of, phenols and, 4
Naltrexone, impact on appetite, 12
National Task Force on the Prevention
 of Obesity, obesity drugs
 and, 113
Native-American children, obesity
 among, 104
Nausea, ginger as remedy for, 56
Negative emotions
 binge eating and, 129
 overeating rationale, 129
Neurotransmitter synthesis
 conditions necessary for diet to
 affect, 36
 enzymes and, 36
Neurotransmitters. *See* 5-HT
New drug application (NDA)
 dietary supplement manufacturers
 and, 80
 health claims and, 73-74
 supplement manufacturers and,
 81-82
Nicotine
 drug dependence disorder and, 18
 effects differ from food, 41
 psychoactive effects of, compared
 with foods, 17
Nitrile compounds, cancer prevention
 and, 3-4
Nonfermented soybean products,
 examples, 53
Nutrients
 bioactive substances in, 1
 pharmacological properties of, 1-16
 types of, 1
Nutrition deficiencies, not common in
 obese individuals, 21
Nutritional supplements. *See also*
 Dietary supplements
 definitions, 66
 sales of, for weight control, 125

OA. *See* Overeaters Anonymous (OA)
Obese binge eaters

normal-weight bulimia nervosa
 patients distinguished from,
 91
 substance abuse and, 92-93
Obese individuals
 addictions model
 promotes deprivation and low
 self-efficacy, 42
 side effects of, 42
 carbohydrate craving and, 88
 control, self-reported lack of, 123
 diets of, neurotransmitter
 biosynthesis alteration and,
 41-42
 implications for treatment, 135-136
 weight fluctuations and, 131
Obesity. *See also* Childhood obesity;
 Obese individuals
 addictions model of, 17,106,143
 management and, 103-104
 pitfalls with, 19-20
 plausibility of, 113
 in adults, medical complications
 and, 105
 behavioral programs for, promising
 results for adults, 111-112
 carbohydrate craving and, 40
 childhood, rates of, 104
 consumption patterns and, 134-135
 control lack
 cultural view of, 124
 reported, 123
 costs of
 health care costs, 103
 health impairment, 103
 psychosocial functioning, 103
 definition, 104
 as drug dependence, 18
 appropriateness of
 characterization, 19
 environmental issue, 110,144
 ephedrine and caffeine (EC), FDA
 concerns regarding, 75-76
 etiology, 104,106,143,144
 environment, 109-110,115
 factors in, 106-110

literature on, 106-107
family factor, 109
medical consequences of, 104
not an eating disorder, 88
OA model of treatment and, 19
physical activity level and, 108-109
prevalence of, 104,123,124
    increasing, 104
psychosocial ramifications of,
        105-106
role of television viewing, 109
stigma against, 124
substance abuse
    distinguished from, 143-144
    similarities, 143-144
symptoms of, 124-125
tryptophan/LNAA ratio and, 38
Obesity rates
    increasing, 104
    treatment programs and, 106
Obesity research, carbohydrate
        craving not valuable concept
        in, 41
Obesity treatments, 106
    abstinence, 114
    addictions model, 115,116
        binge eating and, 113-114
        central tenets lack support, 143
        efficacy unknown, 114
    approaches, 110-111
    behavioral programs, 111-112,115
    continual care model, 112
    control
        eating control, implications, 125
        lack of, implications, 123
    dopamine antagonists and, 132
    environmental approaches, efficacy
        of, 143
    nondieting approaches
        addictions model and, 114-115
        efficacy of, 115
        individuals targeted, 114
    Overeaters Anonymous (OA), 114
    pharmacological interventions,
        adjunct to behavioral
        interventions, 112

public health approaches, efficacy
    of, 143
Opioids, impact of, 12
Opioid peptides, eating behavior and,
        131-132
Organosulfur compounds, effects of, 4-5
Osteoarthritis, dietary supplements
        and, 73
Overeaters Anonymous (OA)
    addictions model of obesity and, 19
    efficacy unknown, 114
    obesity treatment program, 114
    philosophy of, 19
    therapeutic effects, research
        regarding, 114
Overeating
    behavior as response to abnormal
        situation, 125
    as disease, 124 (See also Obesity)
    drug addiction compared with, 130
    excessive appetite
        phenomenological correlates of,
        123
        psychological correlates of, 123
    explanations of
        affective, 129-130
        problems with, 129-130
        situational, 129-130
    positive reinforcement mechanisms
        of, 129
    rationales for, 129
    restrictive dieting and, 128
Overweight binge eaters, Overeaters
        Anonymous groups and, 91

PAH. See Polycyclic aromatic
        hydrocarbons (PAH)
Panax ginseng (ginseng). See Ginseng
Peptides
    effects of, 7
    protein hydrolysis of food system
        proteins and, 7
Perpene lactones, Ginkgo biloba
        extract and, 57-58
Pharmaceutical approaches, adjunctive
        therapy, 136

Pharmaceutical industry
  efficacy in, 70
  fraudulent practices in, regulation
    to prevent, 70
  safety in, 70
Pharmaceuticals. *See also* Dietary
    supplements
  federal regulation of, 70
Pharmacological interventions, obesity
    treatment, 112-113
  drug types, 112-113
Pharmacological properties, of foods,
    141
Pharmacotherapy, for obesity
  attrition rates, 113
  side effects, 113
Phenolic compounds
  effects of, 4
  presence of, 4
Physical activity
  obesity and, 106, 115
  obesity factor, 108-109
Physiological influences, of bioactive
    substances, 2
Pizza, food cravings and, 11
Placebo effect, diet-behavior link and,
    35
Placebo groups, lack of, diet-behavior
    research and, 31,32
Plants for healing, history of, 49-50
Platelet aggregation, garlic and, 55
PMS. *See* Premenstrual syndrome
    (PMS)
Polycyclic aromatic hydrocarbons
    (PAH)
  food preservation procedures and, 6
  tumor development and, 6
Precursor to neurotransmitter, plasma
    levels fluctuating, 36
Premenstrual syndrome (PMS)
  carbohydrate consumption
    memory word recognition and,
      10
    mood and, 10
  increased caloric intake and, 7-8
Protein. *See* Nutrients

Protein hydrolysates, gut hormones
    and, 7
Protein products. *See also* Dietary
    supplements
  dietary supplement, use in US,
    66-67
Protein-rich meals, brain levels of
    tryptophan and, 37-38
Psychoactive substance, distinguished
    from food, 21
Psychosocial consequences, obesity
    and, 105-106
Public health interventions
  eating control, loss of, 125
  obesity treatment and, 143
Public policy
  implications, of biopsychosocial
    model, 136
  obesity and, 123

Quality control, dietary supplements,
    regulatory problems and,
    78-79
Quality standards
  dietary supplements, need for,
    80-81
  drugs and supplements, different
    sets for, 81

Regulations, shortcomings of current,
    78-80
Regulatory agencies in US, food
    classification and, 144
Regulatory impact, foods as drugs and,
    141
Researcher bias, diet-behavior
    research and, 32
Restaurant industry, portion size
    reduction, as public policy
    avenue, 136
Restrictive dieting
  eating control and, 130
  as treatment, avoidance of, 135
Rheumatism, ginger and, 57

Saccharin
 behavioral problems and, 30-31
 compared with sugar, 30-31
Safety, dietary supplements, proof not
  required, 79
Salicin, white willow bark and, 74
Salicylates, aspirin sensitivity and, 23
Sampling problems, diet-behavior
  research and, 31,32
Sassafras
 availability of, 77
 carcinogenicity of, 75,77
 dietary supplement, 66
 efficacy of, 74-75
 prohibited products and, 75
 safety of, 74-75
 uses of, 74-75
  banned, 77
Seasonal affective disorder, vitamin D
  and, 13
Self-medication, problems with, 60-61
Serotonergic neurons, dietary variables
  effect limited by, 39
Serotonergic neurotransmission, drugs
  that increase, carbohydrate
  intake and, 40
Serotonin. *See also* 5-HT
 biosynthesis of, 35
 carbohydrates and, 88
 tryptophan and, dietary, 35
Serotonin release, carbohydrate
  consumption and, 9-10
Serotonin reuptake inhibitors (SSRIs),
  St. John's Wort and, 78,79
Serotonin synthesis, enzymes and, 37
Serum cholesterol
 brain chemistry and, 9
 mood and, 9
Sherley Amendment, Food and Drug
  Act of 1906, 70
Smoking, cigarette, vitamin C
  requirements and, 13
Social situations, happy, overeating
  rationale, 129
Social support, as treatment, emphasis
  on, 135

Soybean products
 cardiovascular disease, protective
  effects against, 54
 categories of, 53
 health promoting effects of, 53
 medicinal qualities, 49,51,53
 nonfermented
  anti-carcinogen effect of, 53
  inhibitory effect on abnormal
  cell growth, 53-54
Species survival, functions necessary
  for, physiological support of,
  126
SSRI. *See* Serotonin reuptake
  inhibitors (SSRIs)
St. John's Wort
 adverse side effects of, 60-61
 antidepressant effects of, 76
 antiviral properties of, 60
 classification of, 77-78
 components of, 76
 contraindications for, 79
 dietary supplement, 66
 as drug, 141
 efficacy of, 76,77
 FDA requirements and, 77-78
 as food, 142
 interaction problems with, 79
 medicinal qualities, 51
 medicinal use of, history of, 59
 metaanalysis of, efficacy of, 59-60
 monoamine oxidase inhibitor
  (MAOI), 79
 mood regulation and, 59
 performance better than placebo,
  59-60
 prescription medicine, 76
 safety of, 76-77
 serotonin reuptake inhibitors
  (SSRIs), 78,79
 studies with, 76
 therapeutic effects, belief in, 58
 wound healing properties of, 59
Standardization, dietary supplements,
  regulatory problems and,
  78-79

Starvation, studies of human, 128
Substance abuse
  eating disorders
    association with, 87,92-96
      reciprocal reinforcement
        theory of, 97
    distinguished from, 87
    patients assesed for eating disorder,
      97-98
    treat before eating disorder,
      recommendation, 98
Sucrose
  behavioral problems and, 30-31
  compared with sugar, 30-31
Sugar
  Attention Deficit Hyperactivity
    Disorder (ADHD) and, 21
  behavior alteration in children
    anecdotal reports, 22
    history of notion, 22-23
  behavior and, methodological flaws
    in research, 31
  behavioral problems
    in children, 28-31
    expectancy effects and, 34
    link unclear, 30-31
    link unsubstantiated, 34
  focus of studies on food influences
    on hyperactivity, 28
  hyperactivity and, 27,29
  in children, no causal
    relationship, 31,143
  link dubious, 33-34
  studies with children, 29-30
  learning disabilities and, 28
  mechanism of effect, 28
Supplement quality control, regulatory
  approach and, 78-79
Supplement standardization,
  regulatory approach and,
  78-79

Tea
  consumption
    cancer prevention and, 51-52

  cardiovascular diseases
    prevention and, 52
    worldwide, 51
  extract
    anti-cholesterolemic activity of,
      52
    constituents, 52
  history of, 51
  tumor inhibitory activities, in in
    vitro investigations, 52
  types, 51
Television viewing
  obesity and, 109
  physical activity level and, 109
Terpenes, effects of, 4
Thalidomide tragedy, regulatory
  impact of, 70
Therapeutic claims, federal regulation
  of, 70
Thio-/Isothiocynates, cancer
  prevention and, 3-4
Tissue extracts. *See also* Dietary
  supplements
  dietary supplement, use in US, 66-67
Toxicity research, need for, 79-80
Toxicologic studies, PAHs and, 6
Trace elements. *See* Nutrients
Trans-fatty acids
  atherogenic quality of, 6
  bioactive substances, 142
Tryptophan
  biosynthesis of 5-HT and, 36-37
  brain levels
    determination of, 37-38
    diets that change, 37-39
  carbohydrates and, 88
  depression and, 35
  dietary, serotonin and, 35
  dietary protein and, 37
  mood regulation and, 35-36
Tryptophan/LNAA ratio
  alteration of, 38
  obesity and, 38
Tumor development, PAHs and, 6
Tumor inhibitory activities, green tea
  consituents and, 52

Tumor-modulating substances, from
    animal products, 5
Twinkie Defense
    sugar blamed for murder, 29
    uncontrollable problem behavior
        and, 29

Uncontrolled studies, diet-behavior
    research and, 31, 32

Vitamin C, cigarette smoking and, 13
Vitamin D, seasonal moods and, 13
Vitamins. *See also* Dietary
        supplements; Nutrients
    deficiencies of
        behavior changes and, 21
        mood changes and, 21
    as dietary supplement, use in US,
        66-67
    Dietary Supplement Health and
        Education Act of 1994 and,
        71
    prevalence of use in US, 66-67
    recommended daily allowances,
        66-67

Water. *See* Nutrients
Weight control, binge eating and,
    90-91
Weight fluctuations, regaining lost
    fat-free mass and, 131
Weight loss
    effective treatments, components
        of, 104
    ephedra, 75
    ephedrine and caffeine, 75
    factors in maintaining, 112
    pharmacological interventions,
        shortcomings associated
        with, 112-113
Weight loss industry
    growth of, 103
    obesity and, 103

Weight loss programs
    behavioral programs, 111-112
    research base of, 111
    variety of, 110-111
Weight management programs,
        continuous care model,
        efficacy of, 136
Weight management treatment
    presenting scenario, 129
    restrictive dieting attempts and, 128
    women in, cultural influences and,
        128
Wheat germ, as dietary supplement, 67
White willow bark
    dietary supplement, 66
    efficacy of, 74,77
    safety of, 74,77
    salicin in, 74
    uses of, traditional, 74
Withdrawal phase, of addiction, 132
Wound healing, St. John's Wort and,
        59

Zingiber officinale (ginger). *See also*
        Ginger
    historical traditions of, 56
    seasoning qualities of, 56

PREVIOUS SPECIAL THEMATIC ISSUES OF ALCOHOLISM TREATMENT QUARTERLY™ ARE AVAILABLE BOUND SEPARATELY

ALCOHOL USE/ABUSE AMONG LATINOS
Issues and Examples of Culturally Competent Services
Edited by Melvin Delgado, PhD
"This book demonstrates how to design and improve services for Latinos with alcohol, tobacco, or other drug problems. . . . The book stresses the importance of cross-cultural knowledge, skills, and community participation."
—Council on Social Work Education
(Alcohol Treatment Quarterly, Vol. 16, Nos. 1/2.)
$49.95 hard. ISBN: 0-7890-0392-9.
$24.95 soft. ISBN: 0-7890-0500-X. 1998. 208 pp. with Index.

SELF-RECOVERY

Treating Addictions Using Transcendental Meditation and Maharishi Ayur-Veda
Edited by David F. O'Connell, PhD, and Charles N. Alexander, PhD
Shows how this ancient system of mind-body medicine, through its mental and physical procedures, can be used to treat addictive diseases effectively.
(Alcoholism Treatment Quarterly, Vol. 11, Nos. 1/2/3/4.)
$59.95 hard. ISBN: 1-56024-454-2.
$24.95 soft. ISBN: 1-56023-044-4. 1994. 524 pp. with Index.

TREATMENT OF THE ADDICTIONS
Applications of Outcome Research for Clinical Management
Edited by Norman S. Miller, MD
"A history and overview of contemporary addictions treatment, detailing informative studies in the field and examining pharmacological and non-pharmacological treatment strategies, treatment effectiveness, and outcome research."
—Sci Tech Book News
(Alcoholism Treatment Quarterly, Vol. 12, No. 2.)
$69.95 hard. ISBN: 1-56024-686-3.
$14.95 soft. ISBN: 1-56023-064-9. 1994. 161 pp. with Index.

TREATMENT OF THE CHEMICALLY DEPENDENT HOMELESS

Theory and Implementation in Fourteen American Projects
Edited by Kendon J. Conrad, PhD, Cheryl I. Hultman, PhD, and John S. Lyons, PhD
"A very useful reference book for anyone seeking to develop their own treatment strategies with this patient group or the homeless mentally ill."
—British Journal of Psychiatry
(Alcoholism Treatment Quarterly, Vol. 10, Nos. 3/4.)
$54.95 hard. ISBN: 1-56024-476-3.
$19.95 soft. ISBN: 1-56023-066-5. 1993. 249 pp. with Index.

Faculty: Many of these titles have been used extensively as textbooks. For your no-risk examination copy, see below.

TREATING ALCOHOLISM AND DRUG ABUSE AMONG HOMELESS MEN AND WOMEN

Take 20% Off Each Book! Special Sale
Nine Community Demonstration Grants
Edited by Milton Argeriou, PhD, and Dennis McCarty, PhD
"Should help those in the field to design better programs and develop realistic time lines for attainment of goals."
—Journal of Psychoactive Drugs
(Alcoholism Treatment Quarterly, Vol. 7, No. 1.)
$54.95 hard. ISBN: 0-86656-992-8. 1990. 164 pp.

THE TREATMENT OF SHAME AND GUILT IN ALCOHOLISM COUNSELING
Edited by Ronald T. Potter-Efron, MSW, PhD, and Patricia S. Potter-Efron, MS, CACD
"Provides important insights into the importance to the recovery process of working through feelings of overwhelming shame and guilt."
—Australian Psychologist
(Alcoholism Treatment Quarterly, Vol. 4, No. 2.)
$54.95 hard. ISBN: 0-86656-718-6.
$19.95 soft. ISBN: 0-86656-941-3. 1989. 215 pp.

CO-DEPENDENCY
Issues in Treatment and Recovery
Edited by Bruce Carruth, PhD, CSAC, and Warner Mendenhall, PhDA
A comprehensive manual for counselors and therapists treating co-dependency.
(Alcoholism Treatment Quarterly, Vol. 6, No. 1.)
$54.95 hard. ISBN: 0-86656-920-0.
$14.95 soft. ISBN: 0-86656-942-1. 1989. 167 pp.

DRUNK DRIVING IN AMERICA
Strategies and Approaches to Treatment
Edited by Stephen K. Valle, ScD, CAC, FACATA
Discusses research, policy, and treatment approaches to one of America's most serious problems—the drunk driver.
(Alcoholism Treatment Quarterly, Vol. 3, No. 2.)
$69.95 hard. ISBN: 0-86656-603-1.
Text price (5+ copies): $24.95. 1986. 176 pp

FACULTY: ORDER YOUR NO-RISK EXAM COPY TODAY!
Send us your exam copy order on your stationery; indicate course title, enrollment, and course start date. We will ship and bill on a 60-day examination basis, and cancel your invoice if you decide to adopt! We will always bill at the lowest available price, such as our special "5+ text price." Please remember to order softcover where available.

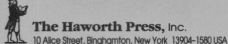

The Haworth Press, Inc.
10 Alice Street, Binghamton, New York 13904-1580 USA

ALCOHOL INTERVENTIONS
Historical and Sociocultural Approaches
Edited by David L. Strug, S. Priyadarsini, PhD,
and Merton M. Hyman
*"A comprehensive and unique account of addictions
treatment of centuries ago."*
—*Federal Probation: A Journal of Correctional Philosophy*
(Monographic supplement No. 1 to Alcoholism Treatment .)
$54.95 hard. ISBN: 0-86656-359-8.
$24.95 soft. ISBN: 0-86656-426-8. 1986. 210 pp. with Index.

PSYCHOSOCIAL ISSUES IN THE
TREATMENT OF ALCOHOLISM
Edited by David Cook, CSW, Christine Fewell, ACSW,
and Shulamith Lala Ashenberg Straussner, ACSW
"Offers approaches to the treatment of alcoholics."
—*The American Journal of Occupational Therapy*
(Alcoholism Treatment Quarterly, Vol. 2, No. 1.)
$69.95 hard. ISBN: 0-86656-363-6.
$24.95 soft. ISBN: 0-86656-401-2. 1985. 134 pp.

CALL OUR TOLL-FREE NUMBER: 1-800-429-6784
US & Canada only / 8am–5pm ET; Monday–Friday
Outside US/Canada: + 607–722–5857
FAX YOUR ORDER TO US: 1-800-895-0582
Outside US/Canada: + 607–771–0012
E-MAIL YOUR ORDER TO US:
getinfo@haworthpressinc.com
VISIT OUR WEB SITE AT:
http://www.haworthpressinc.com

Take 20% Off Each Book!

ALCOHOLISM AND SEXUAL DYSFUNCTION
Issues in Clinical Management
Edited by David J. Powell, PhD
*"A welcome bridge between two disciplines which have
remained separate despite their interrelatedness."*
—*Journal of Sex & Marital Therapy*
(Alcoholism Treatment Quarterly, Vol. 1, No. 3.)
$69.95 hard. ISBN: 0-86656-365-2.
Text price (5+ copies): $24.95. 1984. 135 pp.

Over 250 Pages!

TREATMENT
OF BLACK ALCOHOLICS
Edited by Frances Larry Brisbane, PhD, MSW,
and Maxine Womble, MA
*"Presents some of the outstanding work done
in this area."*
—Dr. Edward R. Smith, Department of Educational
Psychology, University of Wisconsin-Milwaukee
(Alcoholism Treatment Quarterly, Vol. 2, Nos. 3/4.)
$69.95 hard. ISBN: 0-86656-403-9.
Text price (5+ copies): $24.95. 1985. 270 pp.

WE'RE ONLINE!

Visit our online catalog and search
for publications of interest to you by title, author,
keyword, or subject! You'll find descriptions,
reviews, and complete tables of contents
of books and journals!

http://www.haworthpressinc.com

Order Today and Save!

TITLE	ISBN	REGULAR PRICE	20%-OFF PRICE

- Discount available only in US, Canada, and Mexico and not available in conjunction with any other offer.
- Individual orders outside US, Canada, and Mexico must be prepaid by check, credit card, or money order.
- In Canada: Add 7% for GST after postage & handling.
- Outside USA, Canada, and Mexico: Add 20%.
- MN, NY, and OH residents: Add appropriate local sales tax.

Please complete information below or tape your business card in this area.

NAME _____

ADDRESS _____

_____

CITY _____

STATE _____ ZIP _____

COUNTRY _____

COUNTY (NY residents only) _____

TEL _____ FAX _____

E-MAIL _____
May we use your e-mail address for confirmations and other types of information?
( ) Yes ( ) No. We appreciate receiving your e-mail address and fax number.
Haworth would like to e-mail or fax special discount offers to you, as a preferred customer. We will never share, rent, or exchange your e-mail address or fax number. We regard such actions as an invasion of your privacy.

POSTAGE AND HANDLING:	
If your book total is:	Add
up to	$29.95	$5.00
$30.00 – $49.99	$6.00
$50.00 – $69.99	$7.00
$70.00 – $89.99	$8.00
$90.00 – $109.99	$9.00
$110.00 – $129.99	$10.00
$130.00 – $149.99	$11.00
$150.00 and up	$12.00

- US orders will be shipped via UPS; Outside US orders will be shipped via Book Printed Matter. For shipments via other delivery services, contact Haworth for details. Based on US dollars. Booksellers: Call for freight charges. • If paying in Canadian funds, please use the current exchange rate to convert total to Canadian dollars. • Payment in UNESCO coupons welcome. • Please allow 3–4 weeks for delivery after publication.
- Prices and discounts subject to change without notice. • Discount not applicable on books priced under $15.00.

❏ **BILL ME LATER** ($5 service charge will be added).
(Bill-me option is not available on orders outside US/Canada/Mexico. Service charge is waived for booksellers/wholesalers/jobbers.)

Signature _____

❏ **PAYMENT ENCLOSED** _____
(Payment must be in US or Canadian dollars by check or money order drawn on a US or Canadian bank.)

❏ **PLEASE CHARGE TO MY CREDIT CARD:**
❏ AmEx ❏ Diners Club ❏ Discover ❏ Eurocard ❏ JCB ❏ Master Card ❏ Visa

Account # _____ Exp Date _____

Signature _____

May we open a confidential credit card account for you for possible future purchases? ( ) Yes ( ) No

The Haworth Press, Inc.
10 Alice Street, Binghamton, New York 13904-1580 USA

(20) 01/00 BBC00